全国高等中医药院校中药学类专业双语规划教材
Bilingual Planned Textbooks for Chinese Materia Medica Majors in TCM Colleges and Universities

中药化学实验

Experiment Textbook for Chemistry of Chinese Materia Medica

（供中药学类及相关专业使用）
(For Chinese Materia Medica and other related majors)

主　编　高增平

副主编　曲　扬　马　涛

编　者（以姓氏笔画为序）

马　涛（北京中医药大学）
王　薇（陕西中医药大学）
王继彦（长春中医药大学）
曲　扬（辽宁中医药大学）
刘艾娟（北京中医药大学）
李　斌（江西中医药大学）
吴　霞（首都医科大学）
吴锦忠（福建中医药大学）
何永志（天津中医药大学）
何细新（广州中医药大学）
辛　萍（哈尔滨医科大学）
张　薇（北京中医药大学）
邵　晶（甘肃中医药大学）
柴慧芳（贵州中医药大学）
高增平（北京中医药大学）
潘晓丽（成都中医药大学）

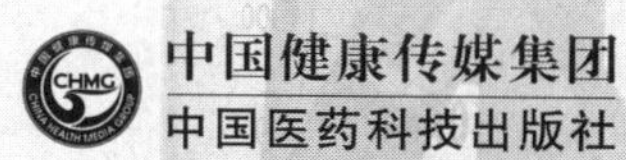

中国健康传媒集团
中国医药科技出版社

内容提要

本教材是“全国高等中医药院校中药学类专业双语规划教材”之一，根据教学大纲的基本要求编写而成，本教材共四章，内容涵盖中药化学实验室规则及安全须知、中药化学成分提取分离及检识方法、预实验方法及实例、主要类型化学成分提取分离及检识的实验实例。实验实例部分通过虎杖、大黄、槐花、补骨脂、防己、黄连、苦参、甘草、薄荷共九味常用中药的提取分离与检识，使学生掌握提取分离及检识的基本操作方法，并加深对理论知识的理解，从而具备从中药中提取分离常见类型化学成分的能力。本教材在附录部分还提供了常用溶剂理化常数表和词汇表，有利于学生了解、选用溶剂和查阅专业英语词汇。

本教材正文部分采用以英文为主、专业词汇在括号内中文标注的方式编写，具有便于通读、易于读懂的特点。在第二、三章及第四章中每一味药实验的开头都有中文“学习目标”，利于学生了解本实验的目的；在结尾都有中文“重点小结”和“目标检测”，利于学生更好地掌握本部分的重点内容，并可针对本实验相关知识进行自行检测，因此本教材具有方便学习、易于掌握重点知识、可自行检测学习效果等实用性强的特点。本教材为书网融合教材，即纸质教材有机融合电子教材、教学配套资源和数字化教学服务（在线教学、在线作业、在线考试）。

本教材可作为全国中医药院校中药学、中药资源学、中药制剂学、临床中药学、中药制药工程等相关专业的本科双语教学、留学生和研究生教学用书，也可作为中医药行业考试与培训及广大中医药工作者参考用书。

图书在版编目（CIP）数据

中药化学实验：汉英对照 / 高增平主编 . — 北京：中国医药科技出版社，2020.8
全国高等中医药院校中药学类专业双语规划教材
ISBN 978 – 7 – 5214 – 1868 – 2

Ⅰ. ①中…　Ⅱ. ①高…　Ⅲ. ①中药化学 – 化学实验 – 双语教学 – 中医学院 – 教材 – 汉、英
Ⅳ. ①R284-33

中国版本图书馆 CIP 数据核字（2020）第 097094 号

美术编辑　陈君杞
版式设计　辰轩文化

出版　**中国健康传媒集团** | 中国医药科技出版社
地址　北京市海淀区文慧园北路甲 22 号
邮编　100082
电话　发行：010 – 62227427　邮购：010 – 62236938
网址　www.cmstp.com
规格　889 × 1194 mm 1/16
印张　6 1/4
字数　161 千字
版次　2020 年 8 月第 1 版
印次　2020 年 8 月第 1 次印刷
印刷　三河市万龙印装有限公司
经销　全国各地新华书店
书号　ISBN 978 – 7 – 5214 – 1868 – 2
定价　29.00 元

获取新书信息、投稿、为图书纠错，请扫码联系我们。

出版说明

近些年随着世界范围的中医药热潮的涌动，来中国学习中医药学的留学生逐年增多，走出国门的中医药学人才也在增加。为了适应中医药国际交流与合作的需要，加快中医药国际化进程，提高来中国留学生和国际班学生的教学质量，满足双语教学的需要和中医药对外交流需求，培养优秀的国际化中医药人才，进一步推动中医药国际化进程，根据教育部、国家中医药管理局、国家药品监督管理局等部门的有关精神，在本套教材建设指导委员会主任委员成都中医药大学彭成教授等专家的指导和顶层设计下，中国医药科技出版社组织全国50余所高等中医药院校及附属医疗机构约420名专家、教师精心编撰了全国高等中医药院校中药学类专业双语规划教材，该套教材即将付梓出版。

本套教材共计23门，主要供全国高等中医药院校中药学类专业教学使用。本套教材定位清晰、特色鲜明，主要体现在以下方面。

一、立足双语教学实际，培养复合应用型人才

本套教材以高校双语教学课程建设要求为依据，以满足国内医药院校开展留学生教学和双语教学的需求为目标，突出中医药文化特色鲜明、中医药专业术语规范的特点，注重培养中医药技能、反映中医药传承和现代研究成果，旨在优化教育质量，培养优秀的国际化中医药人才，推进中医药对外交流。

本套教材建设围绕目前中医药院校本科教育教学改革方向对教材体系进行科学规划、合理设计，坚持以培养创新型和复合型人才为宗旨，以社会需求为导向，以培养适应中药开发、利用、管理、服务等各个领域需求的高素质应用型人才为目标的教材建设思路与原则。

二、遵循教材编写规律，整体优化，紧跟学科发展步伐

本套教材的编写遵循“三基、五性、三特定”的教材编写规律；以“必需、够用”为度；坚持与时俱进，注意吸收新技术和新方法，适当拓展知识面，为学生后续发展奠定必要的基础。实验教材密切结合主干教材内容，体现理实一体，注重培养学生实践技能训练的同时，按照教育部相关精神，增加设计性实验部分，以现实问题作为驱动力来培养学生自主获取和应用新知识的能力，从而培养学生独立思考能力、实验设计能力、实践操作能力和可持续发展能力，满足培养应用型和复合型人才的要求。强调全套教材内容的整体优化，并注重不同教材内容的联系与衔接，避免遗漏和不必要的交叉重复。

三、对接职业资格考试，“教考”“理实”密切融合

本套教材的内容和结构设计紧密对接国家执业中药师职业资格考试大纲要求，实现教学与考试、理论与实践的密切融合，并且在教材编写过程中，吸收具有丰富实践经验的企业人员参与教材的编写，确保教材的内容密切结合应用，更加体现高等教育的实践性和开放性，为学生参加考试和实践工作打下坚实基础。

四、创新教材呈现形式，书网融合，使教与学更便捷更轻松

全套教材为书网融合教材，即纸质教材与数字教材、配套教学资源、题库系统、数字化教学服务有机融合。通过“一书一码”的强关联，为读者提供全免费增值服务。按教材封底的提示激活教材后，读者可通过PC、手机阅读电子教材和配套课程资源（PPT、微课、视频等），并可在线进行同步练习，实时收到答案反馈和解析。同时，读者也可以直接扫描书中二维码，阅读与教材内容关联的课程资源，从而丰富学习体验，使学习更便捷。教师可通过PC在线创建课程，与学生互动，开展在线课程内容定制、布置和批改作业、在线组织考试、讨论与答疑等教学活动，学生通过PC、手机均可实现在线作业、在线考试，提升学习效率，使教与学更轻松。此外，平台尚有数据分析、教学诊断等功能，可为教学研究与管理提供技术和数据支撑。需要特殊说明的是，有些专业基础课程，例如《药理学》等9种教材，起源于西方医学，因篇幅所限，在本次双语教材建设中纸质教材以英语为主，仅将专业词汇对照了中文翻译，同时在中国医药科技出版社数字平台“医药大学堂”上配套了中文电子教材供学生学习参考。

编写出版本套高质量教材，得到了全国知名专家的精心指导和各有关院校领导与编者的大力支持，在此一并表示衷心感谢。希望广大师生在教学中积极使用本套教材和提出宝贵意见，以便修订完善，共同打造精品教材，为促进我国高等中医药院校中药学类专业教育教学改革和人才培养做出积极贡献。

全国高等中医药院校中药学类专业双语规划教材
建设指导委员会

数字化教材编委会

主　编　高增平

副主编　曲　扬　马　涛

编　者　（以姓氏笔画为序）

马　涛（北京中医药大学）　　王　薇（陕西中医药大学）

王继彦（长春中医药大学）　　曲　扬（辽宁中医药大学）

刘艾娟（北京中医药大学）　　李　斌（江西中医药大学）

吴　霞（首都医科大学）　　吴锦忠（福建中医药大学）

何永志（天津中医药大学）　　何细新（广州中医药大学）

辛　萍（哈尔滨医科大学）　　张　薇（北京中医药大学）

邵　晶（甘肃中医药大学）　　柴慧芳（贵州中医药大学）

高增平（北京中医药大学）　　潘晓丽（成都中医药大学）

前　言

中药化学是在中医药基本理论和临床用药经验指导下，运用现代科学理论和技术研究中药化学成分的一门应用学科。中药化学实验是在学习中药化学理论知识的基础上，应用所学理论知识对中药中的化学成分进行提取分离及检识的实践性课程，通过该课程的学习，使学生掌握提取分离及检识的基本操作方法，并加深对理论知识的理解，从而具备从中药中提取分离常见类型化学成分的能力，因此中药化学实验课程，是中药化学理论知识的实际应用，对学生将来从事中药相关领域的工作具有重要意义。

本教材是根据中药学类专业本科中药化学实验课程教学大纲的基本要求编写而成，全书共四章。第一章引言，介绍中药化学实验室规则和安全须知；第二章介绍中药化学成分提取分离及检识的方法；第三章介绍中药化学成分预实验方法和实例；第四章是主要类型化学成分提取分离及检识的实验实例，包括蒽醌类（虎杖、大黄），黄酮类（槐花），香豆素类（补骨脂），生物碱类（防己、黄连、苦参），皂苷类（甘草）和挥发油（薄荷）共九味常用中药，其中苦参为设计性实验，薄荷为挥发油的提取和检识，其余每味中药的实验均包括前言、原理、材料与试剂、实验方法、实验流程、注意事项六个部分；附录包括常用溶剂理化常数表和词汇表，有利于学生了解、选用溶剂和查阅专业英语词汇。

本教材正文部分采用以英文为主、专业词汇在括号内中文标注的方式编写，具有便于通读、易于读懂的特点。在英文部分，坚持语句语法简单化、专业词汇规范化的编写原则，逐句逐词斟酌，以利于教师准确施教，便于学生易学易懂。在第二、三章及第四章中每一味药实验的开头都有中文“学习目标”，利于学生了解本实验的目的；在结尾都有中文“重点小结”和“目标检测”，利于学生更好地掌握本部分的重点内容，并可针对本部分内容的相关知识进行自我检测。本教材为书网融合教材，即纸质教材有机融合电子教材、教学配套资源和数字化教学服务（在线教学、在线作业、在线考试）。

本教材可作为全国中医药院校中药学、中药资源学、中药制剂学、临床中药学、中药制药工程及相关专业的本科双语教学、留学生和研究生教学用书，也可作为中医药行业考试与培训及广大中医药工作者参考用书。

在教材编写过程中，参考、引用了大量文献资料，因篇幅有限仅将主要参考书籍列在全书末尾，参加编写院校的领导和众多专家及同行都给予了热情的鼓励与支持，提出了很多宝贵意见和建议，在此一并表示衷心感谢！

教材编写立足“精品”，各个环节层层严格把关，但是编者水平所限，难免有不妥之处，希望广大师生和读者给予批评指正，以便日后再版时予以完善，使教材质量进一步提升。

编　者

2020 年 3 月

Preface

Chemistry of Chinese Materia Medica is a science that studies the chemical constituents of Chinese materia medica, by using physical, chemical and other modern scientific technologies, under the guidance of the basic theories and clinical experiences of Chinese medicine. The Experiment of Chemistry of Chinese Materia Medica is a practical course to extract, isolate and identify the chemical constituents in Chinese materia medica on the basis of the theoretical knowledge of Chemistry of Chinese Materia Medica. Through the study of this course, students can master the basic operation methods of extraction, isolation and identification, and deepen their understanding of theoretical knowledge, so that they can gain the ability to extract and isolate common types of chemical constituents from Chinese materia medica. Therefore, this experimental course is the practical application of the theoretical knowledge of Chemistry of Chinese Materia Medica, which is of great significance for students to engage in the related fields of Chinese Materia Medica in future.

This textbook is compiled according to the basic requirements of the teaching syllabus of "Experiment of Chemistry of Chinese Materia Medica" for undergraduate students majoring in Chinese Materia Medica. There are four chapters in this textbook. The first chapter is the introduction, which introduces the rules and safety precautions in the laboratory of Chemistry of Chinese Materia Medica. The second chapter introduces the methods of extraction, isolation and identification for chemical constituents in Chinese materia medica. The third chapter introduces the preliminary test methods on chemical constituents from Chinese materia medica and examples are given. The fourth chapter describes the representative experiment examples for extraction, isolation and identification of main types of chemical constituents, including anthraquinones (from Polygoni Cuspidati Rhizoma et Radix and Rhei Radix et Rhizoma), flavonoids (from Sophorae Flos), coumarins (from Psoraleae Fructus), alkaloids (from Stephaniae Tetrandrae Radix, Coptidis Rhizoma and Sophorae Flavescentis Radix), saponins (from Glycyrrhizae Radix et Rhizoma), and volatile oils (from Menthae Haplocalycis Herba). Among the nine commonly used Chinese herbs, Sophorae Flavescentis Radix is selected as the material of a designing experiment and Menthae Haplocalycis Herba is chosen as the material for extraction and identification of volatile oils.The experiments of the other seven Chinese herbs are composed of six parts: Introduction, Principle, Material and Reagents, Methods, Procedure Scheme and Precautions. The appendices of this textbook include a list of physical and chemical constants of frequently used solvents and a related glossary, which are helpful for students to understand the properties so as to select suitable solvents for extraction and isolation, and to consult professional English vocabulary.

The body part of this textbook is mainly written in English, professional vocabulary being marked with Chinese translation in brackets. It is easy to read and understand. In the English part, the principles of sentence grammar simplification and professional vocabulary standardization are preferred. And it is carefully reviewed sentence by sentence and word by word, so as to help teachers teach accurately and students understand easily. The second and third chapters, and each representative experiments in the fourth chapter start with the module of "Learning Objective" in Chinese, which is helpful for students to understand the purpose of the following part; and end with the modules of both "Key Summary" and "Target Detection" in Chinese, which are helpful for students to better grasp the key content of this part and carry out self-test for the relevant knowledge of the experiment. Therefore, this textbook with features of strong practicability is convenient to learn and easy to master key knowledge, and learning effect can be evaluated by self-test. In addition, this textbook is also equipped with digital teaching resources such as courseware and exercise test bank. Students can read the corresponding resources by scanning the two-dimensional code on the paper version of the textbook through their mobile phones, which makes the teaching resources more diversified and multi-dimensional, and realizes the interactive mode of "Book-Mobile terminal-Internet" .

This textbook can be used as the bilingual teaching textbook for undergraduate students, international students and graduate students majoring in Chinese Materia Medica, resource sciences of Chinese materia medica, pharmaceutics of Chinese materia medica, clinical Chinese materia medica, pharmaceutical engineering of Chinese materia medica and other related fields. It can also be a reference book for the examination and training of Chinese materia medica industry and researchers in Chinese Materia Medica.

In the process of compiling the textbook, a large number of literature materials are referenced. Due to the limited space, only the main reference books are listed at the end of textbook. All the leaders, experts and peers participating in the compilation of this textbook provide warm encouragement and support and put forward valuable opinions and suggestions, which are highly appreciated by all editors.

The compilation of the textbook is based on the standard of "High-quality Textbook" . It is strictly controlled from the aspects of compilation, review, editing and publishing. We hope that the teachers, students and readers would give criticism and correction so as to improve the quality of this textbook when it is republished in the future.

Editors

March, 2020

Contents

Chapter 1 Introduction

PPT

The purpose of Chemistry of Chinese Materia Medica (CCMM) experiment teaching is to train students to master the basic skills and knowledge of CCMM, verify the theory of it, and train students to reasonably select the methods for extraction, separation and identification of chemical constituents from Chinese materia medica, as well as the ability to analyze and solve the problems encountered in the experiment. At the same time, experiment is also an important tool to help the student to develop the ability of combining theory with practice, to form the rigorous altitude and good working habits.

Safety is the most important thing during CCMM experiment. Students must learn the laboratory safety precautions first. Before carrying out experiment, students must carefully preview the contents to clarify the purpose and requirements of the experiment, to understand the principles and methods of the experiment, to master the toxicity and other properties of the reagents and remember the precautions in the operation.

Students must abide by the following laboratory rules.

1 Laboratory Rules

1.1 Please wear lab coat.

1.2 Do not be late.

1.3 Take care of all the materials and equipment. Do not take them out of lab without the teacher's permission.

1.4 Keep clean. Wasted organic solvents and caustic liquid should go into the waste jar. No-smoking or eating.

1.5 Preview the contents of experiment and get ready for the materials and the experiment textbook. Check the apparatus in your desk. Let your teacher know if something is broken or missing.

1.6 Strictly follow the experimental procedures to keep safe. Carefully observe experimental phenomenon, take notes, and use your mind. Inform your teacher if the phenomenon of your experiment is abnormal. Return the public apparatus, reagents and materials to the original place after using.

1.7 Clean up your desk and all your tools and put them back when the experiment is over.

1.8 Write your experiment report according to your notes.

2 Laboratory Safety Precautions

Safety is the fundamental guarantee of the chemical experiments. Most of the experimental apparatus are glass. Many of reagents and solvents are flammable, explosive, toxic or corrosive. Improper operation may cause high-risks such as poisoning, fire, explosion, burn, cuts and so on. Therefore, strictly following the procedures and lab rules are very important.

2.1 Prevention of Poisoning

Experimenter should avoid skin or respiratory exposure to toxic reagents to prevent poisoning.

2.1.1 Use an apparatus weighing drugs and reagents.

2.1.2 If you need to smell drugs or reagents to identify, the smell can be slightly smelled far away from the reagent bottle by your hand gently incitement.

2.1.3 The toxic or corrosive gas and volatile liquid should be operated in hood to avoid spread.

2.1.4 If toxic gas was breathed, experimenter should immediately move to outdoor to keep having fresh air. If experimenter's skin touched drugs, water or alcohol can be used to wash. The experimenter should be sent to hospital for treatment if poisoning symptoms appear.

2.2 Prevention of Fire

2.2.1 Volatile reagents should be put in containers with caps or stoppers. Flammable reagents (such as alcohol, ethyl ether, etc.) should be placed far away from the fire.

2.2.2 When the reagent bottle with volatile reagents will be opened, the mouth of the bottle should not be directly set to people's face to prevent suffering harmful gas. Extinguish the fire when combustible liquid is used. If room temperature is high, volatile material should be cooled down before opening.

2.2.3 When volatile and flammable reagents need to be heated, a suitable heat source should be selected.

2.2.4 When volatile and flammable material was distilled, the condenser should be filled with cold water before heating, and it is necessary to keep an eye on the distillation apparatus all the time.

2.2.5 The waste of volatile and flammable materials should be put into special waste containers.

2.2.6 Once the lab catches fire, flammable materials should be immediately removed away from fire, and the source of power should be cut off. Proper types of fire extinguishers should be used. Stone cotton or sands can also be used.

2.3 Prevention of Explosion

2.3.1 Explosion reagents should be preserved at low temperatures and kept away from other flammable reagents.

2.3.2 Do not carry on heating or reactions in a closed system under normal atmospheric pressure.

2.3.3 The exit of high-pressure gas may not face to people. Do not vibrate explosion materials intensely when they are opened or moved.

2.3.4 Experimenters, if necessary, should wear protective masks or explosion-proof screen settings.

2.4 Prevention of Burns

2.4.1 To avoid touching high temperature or corrosive materials, experimenters should wear rubber gloves and protective glasses. To move large bottle of corrosive reagents, it is important to hold the bottle-neck with one hand, and the bottom with the other hand and using mobile carts.

2.4.2 Dilute sulfuric acid in heat-resistant containers, slowly add concentrated sulfuric acid to water and stir constantly with glass rod. Do not add water into sulfuric acid.

2.4.3 Caustic base should be dissolved in heat-resistant container. Strong base and strong acid should be diluted before neutralization.

2.4.4 Burns by acid, wash with 1% sodium carbonate solution, and then wash with water.

2.4.5 Burns by base, wash with 1% boric acid solution, and then wash with water.

2.4.6 Reagents (except of metallic sodium) go into eyes accidentally, immediately rinse with plenty of water.

2.5 Prevention of Cuts

2.5.1 Glass apparatus should be assembled or disassembled gently.

2.5.2 If the joints are not matched, the instrument should not be connected.

2.5.3 If experimenters were injured by glass instruments, glass should be taken out first. The wound should be cleaned and disinfected. If the injury is serious, the injured person should go to hospital.

2.6 Other Safety Precautions

2.6.1 It is important to prevent the sewer from being blocked or corroded. Insoluble solids may not be poured into the sewer. Strong acid, strong base and other poisonous or corrosive liquid should be poured into the sink or should be put into a specific container.

2.6.2 After the experiment, experimenters should shut down the water and the heat, and check the lab for safety.

PPT

Chapter 2 Extraction, Isolation and Identification Methods for Chemical Constituents in Chinese Materia Medica

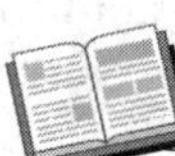

学习目标

知识要求：

1．**掌握** 用溶剂法和水蒸气蒸馏法提取中药化学成分的原理及操作方法；中药化学成分的主要分离方法的原理及操作方法；主要类型化学成分的理化检识反应及薄层色谱显色方法。

2．**熟悉** 常用有机溶剂的性质；常用色谱分离填料的种类及分离原理。

3．**了解** 常用理化检识试剂的组成及配制方法。

能力要求：

能够根据中药化学成分选择合适的提取、分离、检识方法。

To carry on the research of chemical constituents of Chinese materia medica, extraction and isolation of them are the first step.

1 Extraction Methods

The extraction methods include maceration, percolation, decoction, refluxing, and continuous refluxing with solvents. The principle of solvent selection is that those constituents with similar polarity can be dissolved in the solvent. The solvent selection is very important in an extraction method. Among the compound types in Chinese materia medica, the aglycones of terpenoids, steroids and aromatic compounds are less polar, thus can dissolve in organic solvents such as chloroform, ethyl ether, ethyl acetate, *n*-butanol, acetone and ethanol. Glycosides are more polar than their aglycones, thus can dissolve in hydrophilic solvents such as water and ethanol. Compounds with acidic or alkaline functional groups change their state, molecular or ion, in solvent with different pH values, thus their solubility changes based on the pH value of the solvent. The frequently used solvents are listed below according to their polarity from weak to strong.

Petroleum ether (30–60℃ or 60–90℃) < cyclohexane < methylene chloride (CH_2Cl_2) < chloroform

($CHCl_3$) < ethyl ether (Et_2O) < ethyl acetate (EtOAc) < (*n*-BuOH) < acetone (Me_2CO) < ethanol (EtOH), methanol (MeOH) < water (H_2O).

The extraction of effective constituents from Chinese materia medica is more complicated due to the solubilization of multiple constituents. Glycosides and their aglycones both can dissolve in ethanol, so ethanol is the most popular solvent to do extraction. The extraction method is divided into the following means.

1.1 Maceration (浸渍)

1.1.1 Principle of Maceration

Maceration is a process of extracting effective constituents from Chinese materia medica by solvent dissolution and desorption. Generally, this process is divided into solvent permeation, dissolution, desorption, diffusion and replacement. It is suitable for Chinese materia medica with unstable ingredients or high content of starch and mucilage.

1.1.2 Procedures of Maceration

(1) Moisten the Material

Place the properly crushed materials in a covered container, add a proper amount of solvent, stir or shake.

(2) Maceration

Due to the different properties of the materials, the temperature, duration and times of maceration are also different. The specific operations can be divided into cold maceration, hot maceration and re-maceration. At room temperature, the maceration duration may be more than 14days; at 40–60℃, the maceration duration can be shortened, generally 3–7days. During this period, in order to avoid the high concentration of the solution around the material, which is not conducive to the dissolution of the ingredients, the extracted solution should be stirred regularly.

(3) Filter

Pour out the supernatant, filter it, press the residue, combine the filtrate and stand for 24 hours.

1.1.3 Precautions

(1) This method needs large amount of solvent, long extraction time with low efficiency. It is not suitable for the extraction of valuable and toxic materials.

(2) The size of the material should be appropriate, the finer the comminution, the larger the contact area with the extraction solvent, and the faster the extraction speed. However, if the comminution is too fine, the impurities and viscosity will increase, and the filtration will be difficult.

(3) When the solvent is water, the extract is easy to get moldy and deteriorate. It is necessary to add appropriate preservatives.

1.2 Percolation (渗漉)

1.2.1 Principles of Percolation

In the process of percolation, the concentration difference of effective constituents between extraction solvent and percolate always exist, so the extraction efficiency is higher than that of maceration method, which is one of the commonly used extraction methods for thermal unstable chemical constituents.

1.2.2 Procedures of Percolation

(1) Instrument Installation

Fix the iron stand and connect the percolator and collecting bottle in sequence (Figure 2-1).

(2) Moisten the Materials

Place the materials in a suitable container, add equal volume of solvent, mix well, and cover the container. Stand until the materials are evenly moistened, fully expanded and free of dryness.

Figure 2-1 Percolation device

(3) Add Materials into the Percolator

Put appropriate amount of gauze or cotton on the bottom of the percolator, and then put the moistened materials to the percolator. Add a layer of filter paper or cotton on the top of the materials, and add appropriate weight (clean glass ball, etc.) on it to prevent the materials from floating when adding solvent.

(4) Eliminate the Air

Before solvent is added after filling the materials, the air between the materials shall be eliminated as completely as possible, so that the solvent immerses the surface of the materials. Otherwise, the materials are easy to dry and crack, resulting in that when the solvent is added again, it is easy to flow through the cracks, which affects the efficiency.

(5) Maceration

Before percolation, it is usually placed for several minutes to several hours to make the solvent fully permeate and diffuse, especially when preparing high concentration preparations.

(6) Percolation

Generally, the percolation speed is controlled as 1–2 drops per second. When something is extracted in large quantity, the volume of effluent per hour should be equivalent to 1/48–1/24 of the volume of the percolator. If the speed is too fast, the effective constituents will not fully exude and diffuse, and the concentration will be low; if the speed is too slow, the utilization rate of equipment and the experimental efficiency will be affected.

1.2.3 Precautions

(1) The size of the materials should be suitable, too fine to block easily. Although the adsorption is enhanced, the efficiency is low. Coarse materials are not easy to compress, but the contact surface between the solvent and the materials is small, which are not conducive to percolate.

(2) In order to improve the extraction efficiency and avoid the blockage caused by expansion in the percolator, the materials should be macerated by the extraction solvent before it is loaded into the percolator.

1.3 Decoction (煎煮)

1.3.1 Principles of Decoction

There are many kinds of chemical constituents in Chinese materia medica, which interact in the process of decoction, including the physical and chemical changes among constituents, between constituents and solvents. Alkaloids, glycosides, small molecular saccharides, inorganic salts, tannins and other polar constituents are easy to dissolve in water to form a real solution. Most of aglycones, polysaccharides, resins, fats, volatile oils, etc. diffuse out of the plant tissue by heating to form a suspension or colloidal solution. Therefore, the decoction method extracts a wide range of chemical constituents as well as many impurities.

1.3.2 Procedures of Decoction

(1) Maceration

Put the materials into the container, add some water (3–5cm higher than the materials) to macerate. Flowers, stems and leaves should be macerated for 20–30min. Roots, stems, seeds and fruits should be macerated for 60min. The duration can be reduced when the room temperature is high. Do not stay overnight to avoid deterioration.

(2) Decocting

According to the property of the target ingredients, select the appropriate duration of heating gently or strongly. In general, the first decoction is 20–30min, and the second decoction is 10–15min. When the volatile oil is the main active ingredient of the materials, in order to avoid its volatilization, the first and second decocting time should not be too long.

(3) Filtration

The decocted solution is filtered by removing the residue with a filter, and the amount of water added in the second decocting is usually 1/3–1/2 of that in the first time.

1.3.3 Precautions

(1) The decocting containers shall be casseroles (砂锅), pots (陶盆) and enamels (搪瓷), and iron, copper, tin and other metal vessels are forbidden.

(2) To avoid the immediate coagulation of the protein on the surface of the material then affect the dissolution of the effective constituents, cold water is generally used to decoct the drug. However, for the constituents prone to enzymatic hydrolysis, in order to destroy the activity of the enzyme, boiling water can be used to decoct directly.

1.4 Refluxing (回流)

1.4.1 Principles of Refluxing

The refluxing extraction method uses the organic solvent with low boiling point. The solvent is evaporated by heating the flask, and then turns into liquid after condensation (冷凝) and flows back to the flask to extract the materials. The cycle continues until the effective constituents are completely extracted.

1.4.2 Procedures of Refluxing

(1) Sample Preparation and Instrument Installation

Cut the materials into small sections or grind them to appropriate granularity. Add them into the round bottom flask together with the extraction solvent, and install the refluxing device (Figure 2-2).

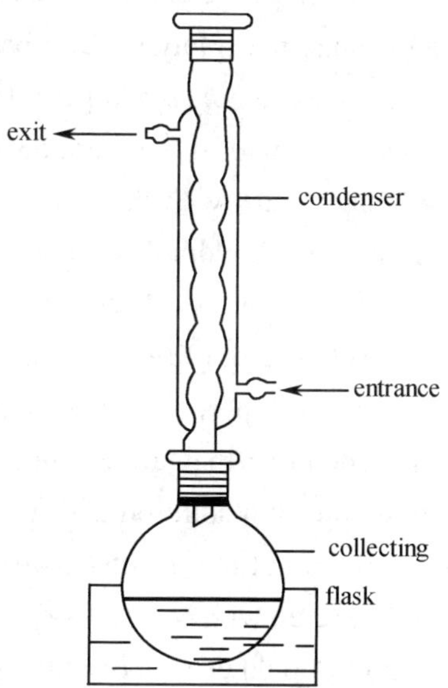

Figure 2-2 Refluxing device

(2) Extraction

Turn on the condensed water and choose a suitable heating apparatus. During extraction, in order to condense the vapor thoroughly, do not boil the liquid excessively. The solvent can be

heated to boil at the beginning of heating, then regulate the heat temperature to make the solvent at a speed of 1-2 drops per second. Generally, the extraction lasts for about 1–3h. Cool down the extracts and filter, add solvent into the residue, and conduct the second and third refluxing. At this time, the refluxing time should be halved until the effective constituents are basically extracted completely.

(3) Concentrated Extract

After the refluxing, remove the heat source first. When there is no condensate drop from the condenser, close the condensing water and remove the device. Combine the extracts. The concentrated extract is obtained by evaporating the solvent.

1.4.3 Precautions

(1) In order to prevent bumping during heating and refluxing, the total amount of solvent is generally 1/2–2/3 of the volume of the round bottom flask. Because there are many pores in the materials, zeolite (沸石) may not be added during extraction.

(2) The order of connecting devices is from bottom to top, and the condensing water flows from bottom to top of the condenser.

(3) Start the timing with the first drop of solvent dropped from the condenser, adjust the heating speed and condensing water flow to control the refluxing speed so that the vapor does not exceed 1/3 of the effective cooling length of the condenser, and pay attention not to interrupt the condensate halfway.

1.5 Successive Refluxing (连续回流)

1.5.1 Principles of Successive Refluxing

The successive refluxing extraction method belongs to the category of liquid-solid extraction, which uses the solvent to evaporate after being heated, and then turns into liquid after being cooled and drops back into the Soxhlet apparatus (索氏提取器), so as to contact the materials for extraction. During this period, through the process of penetration, dissolution and diffusion, the extracted constituents of the materials in the extraction chamber are dissolved and become the solution. When the liquid level of the solvent in the extraction chamber is higher than the upper end of the siphon (虹吸管) in the Soxhlet apparatus, the solution flows back into the round bottom flask. The solution continues to be heated and evaporates, refluxes and percolates, while the solute in the solution remains in the round bottom flask. Therefore, with the extraction process, the solution in the round bottom flask becomes thick, and the solvent contact with the material is fresh. Thus, the ingredients in the materials are gradually transferred to the round bottom flask (Figure 2–3).

1.5.2 Procedures of Successive Reflux

(1) Sample Preparation and Loading

The samples for successive refluxing can be a crude drug or the extract of a crude drug. In the case of crude drug, they are crushed to a certain size. In the case of extract of a crude drug, the extract is first dissolved into solution and mixed with adsorbent such as diatomite (硅藻土), silica gel. The prepared sample is put into a filter paper or a cloth bag, and the height should be 1–2cm lower than the siphon, and covered with cotton. Take care not to leak the sample into the siphon and the round bottom flask. The sample should be packed with appropriate tightness, even and dense.

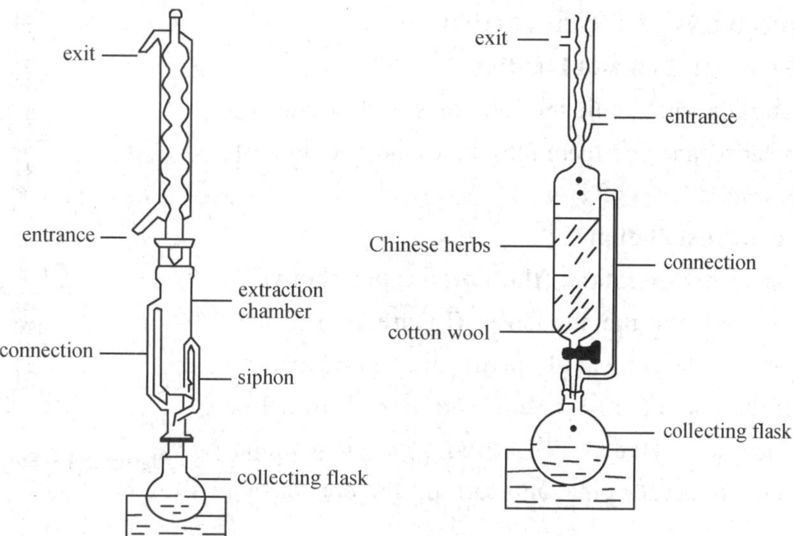

Figure 2-3 Successive refluxing device

(2) Extraction

Add a certain amount of solvent through the extraction chamber, when the liquid level reaches the height of the siphon, it is appropriate to flow into the round bottom flask. Control the heating temperature of the water bath, and control the refluxing speed at 1–2 drops per second.

(3) Concentration

Remove the heat source and let the liquid in the Soxhlet chamber flow into the round bottom flask. Remove the extraction chamber and the samples (including cotton and filter paper). Concentrate the extraction solution in the round bottom flask with distillation device or rotary evaporator to give the extracted substance in the round bottom flask.

1.5.3 Precautions

(1) In order to prevent the constituents from being damaged by heating for a long time, the extract in the round bottom flask can be replaced after extracting for 1–2h with fresh solvent.

(2) The filter paper bag can be made with qualitative filter paper. The height of the filter paper bag should be 1–2cm lower than the siphon of Soxhlet apparatus. The inner diameter of the filter paper bag shall be smaller than that of the extraction chamber. Take care not to leak the materials out the filter paper bag to block the siphon.

(3) In the case of polar gradient extraction, the solvent in the extractor should be evaporated and then replaced with a new solvent for extraction.

1.6 Steam Distillation (水蒸气蒸馏)

1.6.1 Principles of Steam Distillation

Most of the volatile constituents are liposoluble and do not dissolve in water. Under heating, when the sum of the vapor pressure of the two is equal to the atmospheric pressure, the solution begins to boil. The volatile oil can be distilled with water vapor. After the distilled liquid is cooled, the oil layer is separated to obtain the volatile constituents.

1.6.2 Procedures of Steam Distillation

(1) Sample Preparation and Loading

Cut the materials into small sections or smash them into appropriate granularity, and add them into the round bottom flask together with the water.

(2) Instrument Installation

Add a volatile oil extractor (the connection) between the round bottom flask and the condenser (Figure 2-4). If it is necessary to determine the content of volatile oil, add water from the upper end of the volatile oil extractor and make it overflow into the flask, then add xylene (二甲苯) with certain volume. Connect the reflux condenser pipe, and turn on the condensing water.

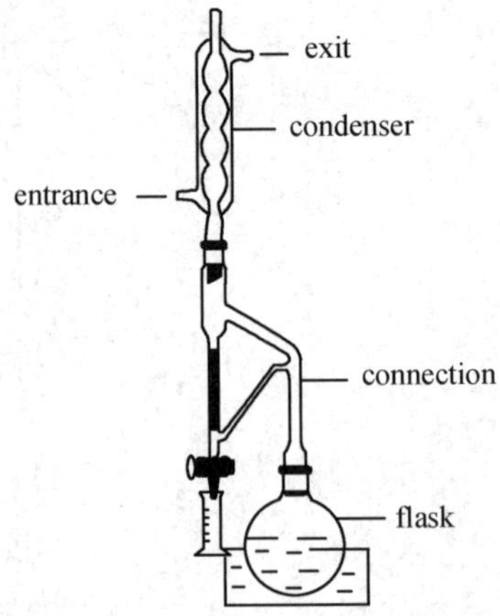

Figure 2-4 Steam distillation device

(3) Extraction

The extraction is the same as that of refluxing method.

(4) Collection of the Volatile Oil

Distill for a period of time until the oil quantity in the graduated tube no longer increases. Stop heating and record the distillation time. Stand for a while, open the faucet (旋塞) at the lower end of the volatile oil extractor, collect the solution. A separatory funnel (分液漏斗) is applied for partition if necessary. The volume of xylene layer in the volatile oil extractor subtract the initial volume yields the amount of volatile oil.

1.6.3 Precautions

The amount of the material used should be large enough to yield no less than 0.5ml volatile oil to preliminarily evaluate the content of the volatile oil in the material by the volatile oil extractor.

2 Isolation Methods

2.1 Crystallization (结晶) and Recrystallization (重结晶)

2.1.1 Principles of Crystallization

The solubility of constituent changes under different temperature. Crystallization is the process that a compound is crystallized from an amorphous form. Recrystallization is the process of crystallization when the primary crystallization is often impure.

2.1.2 Conditions of Crystallization

(1) The concentration and purity of the target compound are high in the mixture.

(2) The key of crystallization method is to choose suitable solvent. The solubility of a compound in an ideal solvent is large at high temperature and small under low temperature. Or in other cases, the solubility of the compound is large in one solvent and small in the other.

(3) Gradually precipitated and crystallized, because impurities might be included when precipitating

suddenly.

(4) Measures to accelerate crystallization include adding seeds, rubbing the inner wall of the container to make scratches, or preparing derivatives.

2.1.3 Precautions

(1) The obtained crystal may be the co-crystallization of compound and solvent molecules. For example, if the solvent is water, it is a hydrous crystal.

(2) In different solvents, the morphology of crystal is different lead to the different melting point. When labeling the melting point of solid compounds, the solvent shall be indicated.

(3) The drying of crystal should be at low temperature, commonly used a vacuum dryer.

2.2 Solvent Precipitation (溶剂沉淀)

2.2.1 Principles of Solvent Precipitation

The principle of solvent precipitation is to change the solubility of constituents by change the polarity or pH value of the solvent. The former includes water extraction and ethanol precipitation, ethanol extraction and water precipitation, ethanol extraction and ethyl ether precipitation, ethanol extraction and acetone precipitation. The latter includes alkali extraction and acid precipitation, acid extraction and alkali precipitation.

2.2.2 Procedures of Solvent Precipitation According to Polarity

There are four types of solvent precipitation according to polarity, i.e., water extraction and ethanol precipitation, ethanol extraction and water precipitation, ethanol extraction and ethyl ether precipitation, ethanol extraction and acetone precipitation.

In the above four methods, the second solvent is added to the solution to change the polarity of the mixture and precipitate some constituents, so as to achieve separation. Several times of high concentration ethanol is added to the concentrated water extract of Chinese materia medica to precipitate and remove water-soluble impurities such as polysaccharides and proteins, and this method is called water extraction and ethanol precipitation. Several times of water is added to the concentrated ethanol extract to precipitate and remove water-insoluble impurities such as resin and chlorophyll, and this method is called ethanol extraction and water precipitation. Several times of ethyl ether or acetone is added to the concentrated ethanol extract to precipitate saponins, while impurities such as fat soluble resin remain in mother liquor.

2.2.3 Procedures of Solvent Precipitation According to pH Values

For acid, alkaline or amphoteric organic compounds, the separation can be realized by adding acid or alkali to adjust the pH value of the solution, changing the existing state of the molecules (free or salt), thus changing the solubility. For example, some alkaloids can be extracted from the Chinese materia medica with acid water and precipitated after the pH of the solution is adjusted to basicity, i.e. acid extraction and alkali precipitation. The method of alkali extraction and acid precipitation is applied to extract acidic compounds such as flavonoids and anthraquinones. To adjust pH value to isoelectric point to make protein precipitate is of the same principle. This method is widely used in industrial production because of its simplicity.

2.3 pH Gradient Partition (pH 梯度萃取)

2.3.1 Principles of pH Gradient Partition

For acid, alkaline and amphoteric compounds, the partition coefficient (K, 分配系数) is affected by the pH value of the solvent system, because changes in pH value can change their state of existence (free or salt), thus affecting the value of K in the solvent system. Therefore, solvent system with organic solvent and buffer solution with different pH value can be used to separate the acidic, alkaline, neutral and amphoteric constituents.

2.3.2 Procedures of pH Gradient Partition

Determination of pH Value of Buffer Solution

① Compounds with Known pK_a Values

Take the acidic compound (HA) as an example. If it is completely dissociated in water, i.e. HA is transformed into A^-, then pH ≌ pK_a + 2; if it is completely free, i.e. A^- is transformed into HA, then pH ≌ pK_a–2. Because pK_a value of phenolic compounds is generally 9.2–10.8, and pK_a value of carboxylic acids is about 5, thus below pH 3 most of the acids will exist in free form (HA), which is easy to participate in organic solvents; while above pH12, they will exist in dissociative form (A^-), which is easy to be participate in water. In the same way, for basic compound (B), when pH is less than 3, it is usually in the form of BH^+, but when pH is above 12, it is in the free form (B).

② Compounds with Unknown pK_a Values

The pK_a value can be obtained by buffer paper chromatography. Take the basic compound as an example. Several buffer strips with different pH value are coated on the filter paper from the high pH value on the starting line to the low pH value, and the solvent system composed of water saturated lipophilic organic solvent is used as the developing agent. In the developing process of the mixture, due to the different basicity, the alkaloids with strong basicity first become salt under the weak acid condition, the polarity becomes larger, and the spots remain at the corresponding strips. Thus the alkaloids are separated by basicity from strong to weak. It is possible that the alkaloids that are not developed at starting line are water-soluble alkaloids. Buffer paper chromatography can be used as the basis for the selection of pH gradient partition conditions of alkaloids.

2.4 Column Chromatography (柱色谱)

Column chromatography is a routine method for the separation of constituents from Chinese materia medica in the laboratory. Generally speaking, non-polar constituents are mainly separated on silica gel, alumina and other adsorption column chromatography, and polar constituents mostly use partition column chromatography for isolation. The separation of acid, alkaline or amphoteric constituents can be achieved on ion-exchange column chromatography. Compounds with large molecular size differences can be separated by using steric exclusion chromatography.

2.4.1 Adsorption Chromatography

(1) Principles of Adsorption Column Chromatography

Adsorption chromatography is one of the most popular chromatography techniques. It involves partitioning of molecules between a solid stationary phase and a liquid mobile phase. The dynamic

equilibrium of solutes as they switch between the stationary phase and mobile phases is specific for each molecule and is affected by competition that exists between solutes and solvents. The separation principle is shown in Figure 2-5.

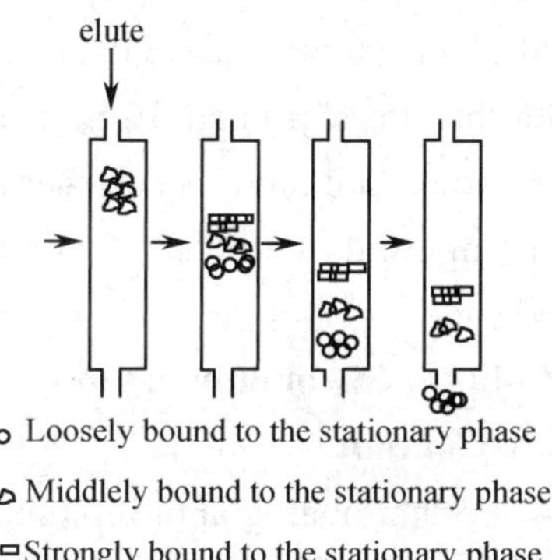

Figure 2-5 Separation principle of adsorption chromatography

The commonly used adsorbents (吸附剂) are alumina, silica gel, polyamide and activated charcoal.

① **Alumina**

Alumina is widely used in the separation of alkaloids, steroids and terpenes. Alumina can be divided into alkaline alumina, neutral alumina, and acidic alumina according to the preparation methods. Among them, neutral alumina is the most widely used. Alkaline alumina is suitable for the separation of neutral and alkaline compounds, while acidic alumina is suitable for the separation of acidic compounds. Some acidic and phenolic compounds are easy to combine with alumina and lead irreversible adsorption. In addition, alumina column chromatography can cause isomerization, oxidation, dehydration and other reactions of some compounds.

② **Silica Gel**

Silica gel is suitable for the separation of quinones, phenylpropanoids, flavonoids, terpenoids, steroids, and other constituents. In addition, silica gel can also be used as a supporting agent for partition chromatography, and can be used for the separation of water-soluble constituents or polar compounds.

③ **Polyamide**

Polyamide molecules contain amide bonds, which can form hydrogen bonds with phenols, carboxylic acids, quinones and other compounds, so as to produce "hydrogen bond adsorption". In addition, in the separation of terpenoids, steroids, alkaloids, sugars and other compounds, polyamide chromatography has a "dual chromatography" performance, that is, there are both non-polar fatty chains and polar amide groups in polyamide molecules. When polar mobile phase (such as aqueous solvent system) is used, polyamide acts as a non-polar stationary phase, and its chromatographic behavior is similar to reversed phase partition chromatography. When non-polar mobile phase (such as chloroform and methanol) is used, polyamide is a polar stationary phase, and its chromatographic behavior is similar to that of normal phase partition chromatography.

④ **Activated Charcoal**

Activated charcoal column chromatography is mainly used for the separation of water-soluble

compounds, such as amino acids, saccharides and some glycosides. In addition, because it is a non-polar adsorbent, it is also commonly used to remove the lipophilic pigment in the extract of Chinese materia medica. The adsorption capacity of activated charcoal is the strongest in water, but weak in organic solvent. Under certain conditions, the adsorption rules of different compounds are as follows:

a. The adsorption capacity of compounds with more polar substituents is higher than that of compounds with less polar substituents. For example, the adsorption capacity of activated charcoal for acidic and basic amino acids is stronger than that for neutral amino acids.

b. The adsorption capacity of aromatic compounds is stronger than that of aliphatic compounds.

c. The adsorption capacity of compounds with large molecular weight is greater than that of compounds with small molecular weight.

(2) Procedures of Adsorption Column Chromatography

① Selection of Chromatographic Column

The ratio of inner diameter to length of chromatographic column is generally between 1 : 10 and 1 : 20. In the case of separating constituents with similar properties, a thin column can be used.

② Packing Column

There are two methods of column packing to give two kinds of column, i.e. wet column and dry column.

a. Wet Column

The requirement of packing a wet column is even filling, and there should be no bubbles. If the column is not even, the moving speed of the compound is irregular, which affects the separation effect. Firstly, take a certain volume of solvent (V_1) and put it into the chromatographic column blocked with cotton, and then take a certain volume of solvent (V_2) to fully swell the adsorbent (alumina can be added directly in the form of powder without swelling). Open the piston (活塞) of the chromatographic column slightly, let the solvent drop into the collecting bottle, add the swelled adsorbent into the column in one time. After adding, discharge all the solvents above the column bed into the collecting bottle, and measure the solvent volume (V_3). Through the equation, $V_1+V_2-V_3$, the column volume of chromatographic is calculated. Therefore, the volume of eluent (洗脱液) and the time to start collecting fractions and to change the eluent are also known.

b. Dry Column

The apparatus used for dry packing include glass column and polyethylene film column. The advantage of glass column is that it is easy to be packed as a more even dry column, but it is not easy to be divided. Because UV light does not penetrate the glass, the position of each band on the column cannot be determined by UV light. It is difficult to pack the column with polyethylene film, but it can overcome the shortcomings of the glass column. Pour the required adsorbent fractions into the column, and after each pour, tighten the column on a hard surface.

③ Loading Sample

There are two ways to load sample.

a. Wet Sample

If the sample can be dissolved in the mobile phase solvent, the sample can be dissolved in a certain volume of solvent. The polarity of the selected solvent should be low, and the volume should be small. Because large volume of solvent often makes the spectral band disperse. Generally, the volume should not exceed the value of the weight of the adsorbent.

b. Dry sample

The sample can also be dissolved with appropriate solvent (note that the amount should not be too large), and then the dry adsorbent such as silica gel is added. Stir until the sample is completely evenly adsorbed on the silica gel. After the volatilization of the solvent, the sample becomes the state of dry fine powder.

④ Elution and Fraction Collection

Add the selected eluent to the adsorption column, release the piston at the lower end of the column and adjust the flow rate. The eluate (洗出液) can be collected by equal amount or by equal time. If there is a means to indicate the color or fluorescent band, it can also be collected according to the color band.

(3) Precautions

① Commonly used columns are glass columns. The specification of the column depends on the compound to be separated. The ratio of inner diameter to column length is generally between 1 ∶ 10 and 1 ∶ 20. If there are special needs, in order to improve the separation efficiency, a thin column can be used. In the case of absorbing some constituents from the solution or filter out insoluble compounds or fine activated charcoal particles when using activated charcoal for decolorization (脱色), a short and thick column can be used. The particle size of adsorbent used for preliminary separation is generally 80–100 mesh, and that for further separation is generally 200–300 mesh. The amount of adsorbent is determined according to the quantity of samples to be separated. If silica gel is used as the stationary phase, the ratio is generally(1 ∶ 30)–(1 ∶ 60). For compounds difficult to separate, the ratio can be as high as(1 ∶ 500)–(1 ∶ 1000).

② During the whole process, the solvent on the adsorbent surface must not be dried, that is, a layer of solvent should be kept on the top of the adsorption column. Once the column solution dries, even the eluent is added, bubbles or cracks often appear in the column, thus affecting the separation.

③ The solvent system of adsorption column chromatography can be screened by TLC. However, because the surface area of the adsorbent used for TLC is generally about 2 times of that used for column chromatography, the solvent system which can make the Rf value of the constituent at 0.2–0.3 in TLC can be selected as the optimal solvent system for column chromatography.

2.4.2 Partition Chromatography

(1) Principles of Partition Column Chromatography

Partition chromatography is to separate compounds with different *K* in two immiscible solvents. A porous substance, such as silica gel, diatomite, fiber powder, microporous polyethylene powder and so on, is often used as a supporter to adsorb a polar solvent, which is always fixed on the supporter during the chromatographic separation process, that is, stationary phase. In addition, it was eluted with a non-polar solvent which was insoluble in the stationary phase. The eluent was always mobile in the chromatographic separation process, i.e. mobile phase. In this system, the polarity of the mobile phase is larger than that of the stationary phase, so it is called reversed phase chromatography. The substance partitioned continuously and dynamically between the stationary phase and the mobile phase on the column, which is separated due to the difference of *K* between the two phases. The difficulty of separation mainly depends on the ratio of the *K*, i.e. separation factor (β,分离因子). If the *K* value is too large, reversed phase partition chromatography can be used, i.e. non-polar solvent as stationary phase and polar solvent as mobile phase. In common use, silica gel is chemically modified and bonded with alkyl groups with different lengths to form lipophilic surfaces. According to the length of alkyl groups, it can be divided into RP-C_2 (ethyl), RP-C_8 (octyl) and RP-C_{18} (octadecyl). At present, reversed stationary phase is commercialized. It can be packed into the column according to the way of adsorption chromatography.

(2) Procedures of Partition Column Chromatography

The operation of the partition chromatography is generally the same as that of the adsorption chromatography. The stationary phase solvent is added to the supporting agent, stirred and mixed evenly, poured into the mobile phase, stirred fully, and the two phases are mutually saturated to reach equilibrium. A small amount of mobile phase is added to the chromatographic column, and the stationary phase is packed in the column. Tap the column gently to let the stationary phase pack evenly. The sample is generally soluble in the mobile phase, eluted with mobile phase, collected according to the fixed volume and concentrated.

(3) Precautions

① In general, the volume ratio of two-phase solvent used in solvent partition is about 1∶1, but the volume of mobile phase in partition chromatography is usually 5–10 times that of stationary phase. Therefore, the *K* value of sample in two-phase solvent should be 0.1–0.2. If the value of *K* is too large, the sample will be eluted from the column quickly and yield poor separation effect.

② The two-phase solvents used must be saturated with each other, otherwise the volume of the stationary phase will change continuously during the separation process, and the partition equilibrium conditions cannot be reached.

③ The ratio of supporter to stationary phase is（1∶0.5）–（1∶1）, that is to say, it is more suitable for silica gel to absorb 50% – 100% stationary phase of its own weight.

④ The ratio of the diameter to the length of the column is（1∶10）–（1∶20）. If the *K* values of the constituents to be separated are close, it can be increased to more than 1∶40. In general, the separation effect of a chromatographic column one-meter long is equivalent to that of hundreds of counter current distribution.

⑤ The ratio of sample to the stationary phase is about（1∶100）–（1∶1000）, which depends on the difficulty of separation. For the constituents with small β value, ratio of 1∶10000 can be used.

⑥ Since the partition coefficient varies with the temperature, for the experiment with higher requirements, it is better to have a spacer sleeve (隔套) to keep the chromatographic column at a constant temperature through water.

2.4.3 Ion Exchange Chromatography

(1) Principles of Ion Exchange Chromatography

Ion exchange resin is used as the stationary phase in the ion exchange chromatography, and the column is packed with water or aqueous solvent. When the mobile phase flows through the exchange column, the neutral molecules in the solution and the compounds that do not exchange with the exchange group of the resin will flow out from the bottom of the column, while the ions in the solution will exchange with the exchange group on the resin and be adsorbed on the column. Then elute the column with appropriate solvent to achieve the separation of compounds.

The appearance of ion exchange resin is spherical particles, insoluble in water, but can expand in water. According to different exchange groups, ion exchange resins are divided into cation (阳离子) and anion (阴离子) exchange resin. The factors affecting ion exchange include pH value of solution, selectivity to exchange ions, concentration of exchanged compound in solution, temperature, and solvent.

① pH value of Solution

Ion exchange can be simply understood as a polymer insoluble acid or base, so the pH value of solution is closely related to ion exchange. When the concentration of hydrogen ion in the exchange solution is significantly increased, the ionization of acidic groups in the cation exchange resin is inhibited due to the common-ion effect, so the ion exchange reaction is seldom or even not carried out. Generally, the pH value of the exchange solution of strong acid cation exchange resin should be greater than 2. Therefore, the pH value of the exchange solution of strong alkaline anion exchange resin should be less than 12, and that of the weak alkaline anion exchange resin should be less than 7.

② Selectivity to Exchange Ions

The adsorption capacity of ion exchange resin to compounds mainly depends on the charge, radius (半径) and acidity or basicity of the dissociated ions. The larger dissociation constant and the stronger acidity or basicity is, the easier to exchange, but the more difficult to elute. The higher the valence (化合价) number of dissociated ions and the larger the charge, the stronger the adsorption and the easier to exchange on the resin. The adsorbability of alkali metals, alkaline earth metals and rare earth elements is also related to their atomic number. When the atomic number is larger, the adsorbability is stronger.

③ Concentration of Exchanged Compound in Solution

Ion exchange is usually carried out in aqueous solution or polar solvent containing water, which is conducive to dissociation and exchange. The solution with low concentration has high selectivity to ion exchange resin. The degree of dissociation tends to decrease at high concentration. Sometimes, it will affect the adsorption order and selectivity; when the concentration is too high, it will also cause the shrink of the resin surface and internal cross-linked mesh, which will affect the entry of ions into the mesh. Therefore, the concentration of the solution used in the general experimental operation should be dilute, which is conducive to extraction and separation.

④ Temperature

The change of temperature has little effect on the exchange performance of dilute solution. But at the concentration above 0.1mol/L, the ions with high hydration tendency are easy to exchange and adsorb with the increase of temperature. At the same time, the activity coefficient of ions increases, which has a great influence on the exchange rate of weak acid and weak alkaline ion exchange resin. Generally, with the increase of temperature and the speed of ion exchange, the elution ability can also be improved. But for the heat-sensitive exchange resin, the increasing of the temperature also leads to the damage of the resin.

⑤ Solvent

Ion exchange chromatography is usually operated in water, as well as in aqueous polar solvent. However, it is difficult to exchange or not to exchange in solvents with small polarity, and the ion selectivity is also reduced or disappears.

In addition, for the exchange resin, if the degree of cross linking is large and the mesh in the resin is small, the large ions can't enter the mesh. Otherwise, if the degree of cross linking is small and the mesh is large, the ion can diffuse and exchange easily. Therefore, the size of the degree of cross linking can increase the selectivity of the exchange resin to the exchanged compound. The size of resin particles will also affect the exchange rate. Small particle size with large surface area is conducive to contact with ions in the solution and increase the exchange rate. Strong acid and strong alkaline exchange resins have strong dissociation ability, so they are easy to exchange with ions in solution.

(2) Procedures of Ion Exchange Chromatography

Ion exchange is usually carried out in a column. Because the samples flowing down the column contact the new resin one after another, there is no reverse exchange. If there are more than two kinds of ions, the different exchange capacity is used to separate the constituents.

① Resin Pretreatment

Pretreatment is an indispensable step before using ion exchange resins. General resins contain soluble small molecular organic compounds and impurities such as iron and calcium. Therefore, pretreatment is needed to remove impurities before ion exchange.

First, the new resin was immersed in distilled water for 1-2 days to fully expand. According to the properties of the exchange group of the resin, carry out the following operations (See a-d).

a. Strong Acidic Cation Exchange Resin

The cation on new resin is generally Na^+. Firstly, 2mol/L hydrochloric acid with 20 times of resin volume is exchanged at a speed of about 1ml/min to exchange the cation to H^+, then wash the resin with water until the eluate is neutral, and then wash the resin with 1mol/L NaOH or NaCl with 10 times of resin volume to exchange the cation to Na^+. Wash with water until the eluate does not contain Na^+ (flame reaction can be applied to identify). Repeat hydrochloric acid to sodium hydroxide (or sodium chloride) treatment again. Finally, 1mol/L hydrochloric acid solution with 10 times of the resin volume is used to exchange the cation to H^+, and then distilled water is used to wash until the eluate is neutral.

b. Strong Basic Anion Exchange Resin

The anion on new resin is generally Cl^-. Firstly, use 20 times of the resin volume 1mol/L NaOH solution to change the anion to OH^-, and use 10 times of the resin volume of water to wash. Then, the resin is changed into Cl^- type by 10 times of the volume of 1mol/L hydrochloric acid solution. Wash with distilled water to near neutral. Repeat sodium hydroxide to hydrochloric acid treatment again. Finally, 1mol/L NaOH solution with 10 times the volume of the resin is used to exchange the anion to OH^-. OH^- type resin is easy to absorb carbon dioxide in the air, so it should be noted that it is better to change Cl^- type resin into OH^- type resin before use.

c. Weak Acidic Cation Exchange Resin

The cation on new resin is generally Na^+. Firstly, the cation on the resin is changed to H^+ type with 1mol/L hydrochloric acid solution 10 times of the resin volume. Wash with water until the eluate is neutral. Then, the 1mol/L sodium hydroxide solution with 10 times of the resin volume is used to change it to Na^+, at this time, the volume of the resin expands. Wash with water 10 times the volume of resin. The eluate is still weakly alkaline. Repeat hydrochloric acid to sodium hydroxide treatment again. The resin is changed to H^+ type with 1mol/L hydrochloric acid solution 10 times the volume of resin. Wash to neutral with water.

d. Weak Basic Anion Exchange Resin

The anion on new resin is generally Cl^-. The pretreatment is the same as the strong basic anion exchange resin. It is not easy to wash it to neutral because of hydrolysis. Generally, water with 10 times the volume of resin is used.

In addition to hydrochloric acid, sulfuric acid is sometimes used. And ammonium chloride can be used instead of sodium chloride.

② Packing Ion Exchange Resin Column

Put the resin in the beaker, add water and stir fully to drive out the bubbles. Stand for a few minutes to allow most of the resin to settle and remove the cracked particles. Repeat the above operation until the supernatant (上清液) is transparent.

Put some cotton at the bottom of column, and press it flat with glass rod. Stir the resin with a small amount of water, and then pour it into the column which is vertical to make the resin settle. Try to finish the packing at one time. Otherwise, the resin with larger particle size range will be layered in the process of pouring for many times, leading the particle size at the upper and lower parts of the column inconsistent. In addition, do not let bubbles enter into the resin layer to avoid uneven contact between the sample solution and the resin. The solution level is kept above the resin layer. When adding the solution, pay attention not to disperse the resin.

③ Sample Loading

Each resin has a certain exchange equivalent. For cation exchange resin, the sample can be added to 1/2 of the total exchange equivalent. And for anion exchange resin, the sample can be added to 1/4 –1/3 of the total exchange equivalent.

④ Elution

For the cation exchange resin with exchanged alkaloids, the alkali solution [such as 10% ammonia (氨水)] is used for alkalization, and then organic solvents such as ethyl ether, chloroform, methanol are used for elution to yield the total alkaloids. Or add acidic water or basic ethanol to elute the resin to obtain alkaloid salt or free alkaloid respectively. For the anion exchange resin with exchanged acidic compounds, the resin can be eluted with acidic ethanol or basic water to obtain the acidic compounds in free and salts forms respectively.

2.4.4 Size Exclusion Chromatography (SEC)

(1) Principles of Size Exclusion Chromatography

Size exclusion chromatography is based on the size of the separated constituents. The stationary phase is a porous filler gel, so it is also known as gel filtration chromatography. The separation mechanism of size exclusion chromatography depends only on the relationship between the pore size of the gel and the size of the separated compound. It has no relation to the nature of the mobile phase, and its function is similar to that of the molecular sieve. In the process of elution, smaller molecules infiltrate into the gel, and larger molecules flow with the solution, depending on the size of the molecule. Therefore, when the chromatographic separation of various constituents is carried out, the order of outflow from the column is arranged in the order of decreasing molecular weight. It is shown in Figure 2-6.

Figure 2-6 Separation principle of SEC

(2) Procedures of Size Exclusion Chromatography

① Selection of Gel

In general, if the constituents to be separated are with extremely different molecular weight, the particle size of gel can be 100–150 mesh. With slow elution, the isolation is achieved. Generally, G-25 is suitable for desalting. But for the samples with close molecular weight, which are easy to overlap between the elution curves, suitable gel types are needed. Sometimes the commercial gels need further treatment. The monomer, powder and fragment of gel are removed by flotation. Gel with particle size of 200 mesh can be selected. The selected gels are swollen in the eluent to be used, and the swelling time varied with the type of gel.

② **Apparatuses**

For primary separation, the column height can be about 30cm, and the diameter of the column is about 2.5cm. When the separation needs to be improved, thin and long columns can be selected. The column height can be up to 1–1.5m. If the sieve plate is installed at the bottom of the column, the space below the sieve plate should be as small as possible to reduce the diffusion of the sample and avoid tailing. In order to make the column bed installed evenly, it is required to install the column once.

③ **Column Packing**

First, fix the column vertically, add a small amount of eluent in the column, and discharge the air under the sieve plate. Tighten the piston, add the eluent to 1/4 the column length, and then add the degassed gel from the top. Open the piston and control the flow rate so that the gel will settle. The flow rate of the column over a meter high is very slow. After all the gel is settled, stand for a while until the surface of the column no longer drop. If the surface of the column is not smooth or the gel particles are adhered to the inner wall of the column, stir the solution 2cm above the column bed gently so that the gel can be suspended and then settled.

Whether the gel column is uniform has a decisive effect on the separation effect. The easiest way to detect the column is to observe whether there is "bubble". A lamp parallel to the column can be placed on the column background for observation. More accurately calibrating the uniformity of the column is the use of colored substances completely excluded by gel, such as blue dextran (葡聚糖) 2000 and cytochrome C. Blue dextran 2000 is commonly used, with an average molecular weight of 2000. Prepare the concentration of 0.2% with 0.02mol/L sodium chloride solution. Add the dye to the top of the column, elute with 0.02mol/L sodium chloride solution, and collect the eluate until the dye starts to flow out. The collected solution is the volume of the column (V_0). In this process, we can know the uniformity of the column from the movement of the blue zone.

④ **Sample Loading**

The gel column should be balanced with at least 3 times the volume of the eluate. After the equilibrium, leave the liquid surface 1–2mm above the surface of the column bed, and the sample will be loaded by the dropper. The sample should be filtered or centrifuged before loading. After adding, open the piston to make the sample completely percolate into the column. Close the piston again, use a small amount of eluent to wash the residual sample on the column wall, open the piston again, until the solution on the top percolate into the column, close the piston, cover the column bed with a thin layer of cotton to protect the surface of the column bed, then add the eluent, and connect the storage bottle.

The volume of sample solution should be small and concentrated as much as possible, so that the outflow peak pattern is normal distribution. For the preparative separation, the sample volume can be larger up to one quarter of the column volume.

⑤ **Elution**

The choice of eluent depends on the properties of the sample. For neutral compounds, the eluents are mostly water and electrolyte (电解质) solutions, such as acid, alkali, salt solutions, and buffer solutions. For the constituents with strong retention, water and organic solvent mixture can be used, such as water-methanol, water-ethanol, water-acetone and so on. Aromatic compounds are strongly retained when they are separated on high crosslinking gel. This effect is weakened or eliminated by different eluent. If the molecular weight of the peptide is determined by cross-linked dextran G-25, the aromatic peptide will not be retained when phenol-acetic acid-water (1 : 1 : 1, w/volume/volume) is used as eluent. Similarly,

sodium hydroxide solution or acetic acid-pyridine buffer, urea (尿素) and potassium thiocyanate (硫氰酸盐) can eliminate the influence of aromatic groups.

⑥ Collection and Detection

Since the flow rate of gel column is slow and there are many fractions collected, it is best connected to the collector and detected according to the characteristics of the separated compound. If the sample is a protein, nucleotide or polypeptide, it needs to be detected by ultraviolet spectrophotometer, and the optical density of each fraction is measured at 280nm, 260nm and 230nm, respectively. Then the elution curve of each constituent is drawn with the sample number as abscissa (横坐标) and the optical density value as ordinate (纵坐标).

⑦ Concentration and Drying of Samples

The fraction of aqueous solution separated by gel chromatography is freeze-dried (冷冻干燥) if it is thermally unstable. If it is a thermal stable compound, it can be heated and concentrated. Fractions containing organic solvents separated by gel chromatography are generally concentrated by vacuum distillation.

⑧ Gel Regeneration

Once the gel column has been used, it can be used again after getting balanced with the buffer. However, if some contaminants are deposited on the surface of the column bed or the gel changes color, this part of the gel can be scraped away with a scraper and properly added with new swollen gel to balance. If the whole column is contaminated, the gel should be regenerated and repacked. The regeneration method is as follows. Immerse the gel with mixture of 0.5mol/L sodium hydroxide and 0.5mol/L sodium chloride at about 50℃, and then wash it with water. The gel is kept in wet state and added 0.02% sodium azide (叠氮化物) to keep it from moldy. If it is not used for a long time, the regenerated gel can be washed with plenty of water, and then gradually increase the concentration of alcohol, so that it will gradually shrink. Then dry at 60 – 80℃, or wash with ethyl ether for quick drying. The distilled water, apparatuses and experimental table used during operation should be clean and free from dust, so as to avoid polluting the gel again.

3 Physicochemical Identification

3.1 Identification Reagents

The fractions obtained by various separation methods are usually identified qualitatively by tube reaction or thin layer chromatography, and the structural types of compounds can be preliminarily determined according to the types of reaction reagents. The reagents used in the identification of chemical constituents in Chinese materia medica are listed as follows.

3.1.1 Universal Chromogenic Reagents

(1) Iodine

Iodine is used to detect of organic compounds. Iodine vapor can make many compounds turn yellow brown. Put iodine into a closed glass container first, so that the air in the container is saturated with iodine vapor.

Put the developed thin-layer plate or paper into the container for several minutes to develop color. Sometimes put a small cup of water in the container to increase the humidity, which can improve the sensitivity.

(2) Sulfuric Acid

10% sulfuric acid ethanol solution reacts with most of the organic compounds to generate colorful products.

3.1.2 Detective Reagents for Alkaloids

(1) Dragendörff Reagent

This reagent is composed of bismuth potassium iodide (碘化铋钾), glacial acetic acid, and water (7.3 : 10 : 60, w/v/v).

(2) Wagner Reagent

This reagent is composed of iodine, potassium iodide (碘化钾), glacial acetic acid, and water (1 : 10 : 2 : 100, w/w/v/v).

(3) Silicotungstic Acid (硅钨酸) Reagent

Silicotungstic acid (5g) is dissolved in 100ml water, and adjusted to pH2 with hydrochloric acid.

(4) Picric Acid (苦味酸) Reagent

This reagent is 1% picric acid aqueous solution.

(5) Tannic Acid (鞣酸) Reagent

Tannic acid (1g) dissolved in 1ml ethanol then add water to 10ml.

(6) Cerium Sulfate (硫酸铈) Reagent

Suspend 0.1g cerium sulfate in 4ml water, then 1g trichloroacetic acid followed by boiling. The mixture is added sulfuric acid until transparent.

3.1.3 Detective Reagents for Saccharides

(1) Fehiling Reagent

This reagent composed of two solutions mixed with equal volume before use. One is 6.23% copper sulphate aqueous solution, and the other is composed of potassium sodium tartrate (酒石酸钾钠), sodium hydroxide, and water (34.6 : 10 : 100, w/w/v). It is used to detect reducing sugar.

(2) Silver Nitrate-Ammonia Reagent

Dissolve 1g silver nitrate with 20ml water, then add ammonia water with stirring until the sediments produced nearly dissolve. The filtrate is used to detect reducing sugar.

(3) Keller-Kiliani Reagent

This reagent is composed of 1% $FeCl_3$ solution and glacial acetic acid (1 : 200, v/v). Dissolve the sample in this reagent. Then add concentrated sulfuric acid along the test tube wall to let the sulfuric acid down to the bottom of the tube. The color change of the acetic acid layer is produced by 2-deoxy sugar. And the color change of the interface originates from the dehydration of aglycone by concentrated sulfuric acid. The color of the interface can be green, red, or yellow-brown based on the structure of the aglycone. It is used to detect 2-deoxy sugar.

(4) Xanthydrol (咕吨氢醇) Reagent

It is the glacial acetic acid solution of xanthydrol with concentration of 0.1mg/ml. It is used to detect 2-deoxy sugar.

3.1.4 Detective Reagents for Glycosides

(1) Molish Reagent

This reagent is composed of 15% α-naphthol ethanol solution, concentrated sulfuric acid, ethanol, and water (21 : 13 : 87 : 8, v/v/v/v). After baking the sprayed TLC at 100℃ for 3–6min, most saccharides and glycosides turn blue, and rhamnose turns orange.

(2) Phthalic Acid (邻苯二甲酸) -Aniline (苯胺) Reagent

Dissolve phthalic acid (0.93g) and aniline (1.66g) in water saturated butanol. After baking the sprayed TLC at 105–110℃ for 5min, most saccharides turn brown.

3.1.5 Detective Reagents for Phenols

(1) Ferric Chloride Reagent

It can be 5% aqueous or ethanol solution of ferric chloride.

(2) Ferric Chloride-Potassium Ferricyanide Reagent

This reagent is composed of 2% aqueous solution of ferric chloride and 1% aqueous solution of potassium ferricyanide mixed with equal volume before use.

(3) Emerson Reagent

This reagent is composed of 2% ethanol solution of 4-aminoantipyrine (安替比林) and 3% aqueous solution of potassium ferricyanide. It is used to confirm whether the *para*-position of phenolic hydroxyl group is substituted. If there is no substitute group on the *para*-position, then the reaction is positive. When there is substitute group on the *para*-position, this reaction is negative.

(4) Gibb's Reagent

This reagent is composed of 0.5% ethanol solution of 2, 6-dichloroquinone-4- chloroimide (2, 6-二氯苯醌 -4- 氯亚胺) and buffer solution containing boric acid (硼酸), potassium chloride, potassium hydroxide (pH9.4). It is also used to confirm whether the *para*-position of phenolic hydroxyl group is substituted. If there is no substitute group on the *para*-position, then the reaction is positive. When there is substitute group on the *para*-position, this reaction is negative.

3.1.6 Detective Reagents for Lactone and Coumarins

(1) Ferric Hydroxamate (异羟肟酸铁) Reagent

Solution a: 1mol/L methanol solution of **hydroxylamine hydrochloride (盐酸羟胺)** prepared before use.

Solution b: 1.1mol/L methanol solution of potassium hydroxide.

Solution c: ferric chloride dissolved in 1% hydrochloric acid with concentration of 1% (w/v).

These solutions are added to the sample solution in the order of a, b, c.

(2) Ring Open-Cycle Reagent

Solution a: 1% sodium hydroxide solution.

Solution b: 2% hydrochloric acid solution.

3.1.7 Detective Reagents for Flavonoids

(1) Hydrochloric Acid-Magnesium Reaction

This reagent is used to detect flavone (黄酮), flavonol (黄酮醇), dihydroflavone (flavanone, 二氢黄酮), dihydroflavonol (flavanonol, 二氢黄酮醇). And chalcone (查尔酮), aurone (橙酮), catechin (儿茶素) do not react. The reagents are concentrated hydrochloric acid and magnesium powder.

(2) Aluminum Trichloride Reagent

This reagent is used to verify whether there is *o*-diphenol hydroxyl or 3-OH, 4-keto or 5-OH, 4-keto moieties in the structure of flavonoids. The reagent is 2% aluminum trichloride methanol solution.

(3) Magnesium Acetate Reagent

The reagent is 1% magnesium acetate methanol solution. This reaction can be carried out on filter paper. During the test, add a drop of test solution on the filter paper, spray with the methanol solution of magnesium acetate, heat and dry, and observe under the ultraviolet light. Dihydroflavone and dihydroflavonol can show blue fluorescence. If they have 5-OH, the color is more obvious. The color of flavonoids, flavonols and isoflavones are yellow, orange or brown.

(4) Basic Lead Acetate Reagent

The reagent is an aqueous solution of saturated basic lead acetate (or saturated lead acetate). It can produce yellow to red precipitate. The color of the precipitation of flavonoids and lead salts varies with the number and position of hydroxyl groups. Among them, lead acetate can only react with compounds with *o*-diphenol hydroxyl or 3-OH, 4-keto or 5-OH, 4-keto structure to form precipitates. However, the precipitation capacity of basic lead acetate is much larger, and the common phenolic compounds can also precipitate.

(5) Potassium Hydroxide Reagent

It is 10% potassium hydroxide aqueous solution.

(6) Zirconium Oxychloride (氯化氧锆) Reagent

The reagents are 2% zirconium oxychloride methanol solution and 2% citric acid methanol solution. When there is free 3- or 5-OH in the flavonoid molecule, it can react with the reagent to form a yellow zirconium complex. But the two zirconium complexes have different stability to acid. The stability of 3-OH, 4-keto complex is stronger than that of 5-OH, 4-keto complex (except for flavanones). Therefore, when citric acid was added to the solution, the yellow solution of 5-hydroxyflavone was significantly faded, while the yellow solution of 3-hydroxyflavone was still bright yellow.

3.1.8 Detective Reagents for Anthraquinones

(1) Potassium Hydroxide Reagent

This reagent is used to identify hydroxyl anthraquinones. The reagent is 10% potassium hydroxide aqueous solution.

(2) Magnesium Acetate Reagent

The anthraquinone with α-hydroxyl and/or *o*-dihydroxyl are identified. The reagent is 10% magnesium acetate methanol solution.

(3) 1% Boric Acid Reagent

Anthraquinone with α-hydroxyl and/or *o*-dihydroxyl are identified. The reagent is 1% boric acid aqueous solution.

3.1.9 Detective Reagents for Cardiac Glycosides

(1) Kedde Reagent

Mix 2% 3, 5-dinitrobenzoic acid methanol solution with 1mol/L potassium hydroxide methanol solution in equal amount. Cardenolide glycosides can be detected.

(2) Baljet Reagent

Mix 1% picric acid aqueous solution and 10% sodium hydroxide solution in equal amount together. Cardenolide glycosides can be detected.

(3) Legal Reagent

It is composed of equal amount of pyridine, 0.5% nitroferrocyanatum natrium, and 10% sodium hydroxide solution mixed before use. This reagent is also used to detect cardenolide glycosides.

3.1.10 Detective Reagents for Saponins

(1) Hemolysis Test

This test needs 2% normal saline suspension of blood cells. The preparation of this reagent is as

follows. Appropriate amount of fresh rabbit blood (blood taken from the heart or ear vein), quickly stir with a clean small brush, remove fibrin and use normal saline to repeatedly centrifugal wash the supernatant. After the supernatant is colorless, measure the settling red blood cells and use normal saline to prepare 2% suspension, and store it in the refrigerator for standby (storage period of 2–3days).

(2) Liebermann Burchard Reagent

The reagent is composed of acetic anhydride and concentrated sulfuric acid.

3.1.11 Detective Reagents for Terpenoids and Steroids

(1) Vanillin-Concentrated Sulfuric Acid Reagent

This reagent is composed of 5% vanillin dissolved in concentrated sulfuric acid solution [or 0.5g vanillin dissolved in 100ml sulfuric acid ethanol (4 : 1, v/v)].

(2) Kahlenberg Reagent

Dissolve antimony pentachloride (五氯化锑) in chloroform (or carbon tetrachloride) with the ratio of 1 : 4, prepare before use.

(3) Liebermann Burchard Reagent

The preparation method is the same as mentioned above in 3.1.10 (2).

(4) Chloroform-Concentrated Sulfuric Acid Reagent

Dissolve the sample in chloroform. Then add concentrated sulfuric acid.

(5) Trichloroacetic Acid Reagent

Dissolve 3.3g of trichloroacetic acid in 10ml of chloroform, and add 1-2 drops of hydrogen peroxide.

3.2 Thin Layer Chromatography (TLC, 薄层色谱)

3.2.1 Principle of TLC

Thin layer chromatography is a method of evenly spreading adsorbent or supporter on the plate to form a thin layer. The sample is spotted on the thin layer, and developed with appropriate solvent to separate it. It is often used to judge the purity of compounds, to separate, purify and determine the content of mixtures, and to explore and determine the elution conditions of column chromatography.

The sample is separated in the adsorbent (stationary phase) by developing solvent on the thin-layer plate. Due to the different adsorption capacity of various compounds, when the solvent develops, the compounds are dissociated and adsorbed in different degrees, so as to achieve the purpose of separation. The specific process is that when the sample contacts the adsorbent, it is adsorbed by the adsorbent, and then when the developing solvent contacts the adsorbent, it rises due to the capillary action, and contacts the sample spots, so that the compound can be desorbed from the adsorbent and dissolved in the developing solvent. When the compound moves with the developing solvent, it meets a new adsorbent, and re-adsorbs. The compounds in the sample are different in the process of adsorption and desorption, and thus to achieve the purpose of separation. Adsorbents used in column chromatography, such as alumina, silica gel, polyamide, etc., can be used in thin-layer chromatography, among which silica gel is widely used for the separation of various compounds due to its good adsorption performance. The selection of adsorbent is mainly based on the solubility, acidity, basicity and polarity of the sample. Alumina is generally an adsorbent with weak basicity, which is suitable for the separation of alkaline and neutral compounds, especially for the separation of alkaloids. Silica gel is an adsorbent with weak acidity, which is suitable for the separation of acidic compounds and neutral compounds. Polyamide can form

reversible hydrogen bond with compounds containing phenolic hydroxyl and carbonyl groups, so it is suitable for the separation of flavonoids and anthraquinones.

3.2.2 Procedures of TLC

(1) Preparing the Thin Layer Plate

Spread the adsorbent or supporting agent evenly on the glass plate to make it a thin layer with a certain thickness. The size of the glass plate can be determined according to the aims of separation. Before preparing the plate, the glass shall be soaked with detergent, and then washed with distilled water. There shall be no oil stain on the glass. Otherwise, the adsorbent cannot be well distributed on the glass.

There are two main forms of plate: one is soft plate, and the other is hard plate.

① Soft Plate

Take a glass rod with a diameter of 1cm, and wrap several circles of adhesive tape around both ends of the glass rod. The thickness is the same with that of the thin layer, which can be determined according to the needs. Generally, the thickness used for identification or quantification is 0.25–0.5mm, the thickness used for small-scale preparation is 1–3mm. The activated adsorbent is poured on the glass plate, one side of the glass plate is fixed, and then the adsorbent is pushed from one side to the other side by pressing the glass rod on the glass plate, forming a thin layer.

② Hard Plate

Add a proper amount of water or adhesive (黏合剂) to the adsorbent to make a paste, then pour it on the glass plate, and make it into a uniform thin layer through the applicator (涂敷器). It can also be laid by hand, that is to say, pour a proper amount of prepared adsorbent onto the glass plate, spread it evenly with a glass rod, tap the glass plate gently to make the surface flat and smooth, and then place it on the horizontal platform. After air drying, activate it in the oven.

(2) Sample Application

Dissolve the tested sample in a small amount of solvent to prepare a 5% solution, and dilute it to a concentration of 1% – 0.01% when using. Generally, volatile organic solvent is selected as the developing solvent in combination with the solubility of the compound, and water is not used as the developing solvent as much as possible, otherwise the spots are easy to diffuse. When apply the sample, capillary or quantitative capillary shall be used, dropping in several times to avoid excessive diameter of the original spot. The size of the spot shall be controlled within 3mm of the diameter, and the spot shall be about 1.5cm from the bottom of the glass plate. If more than one sample is applied on the thin layer, the distance between each sample is about 0.5–1cm, and the origin of each sample should be on the same horizontal line.

(3) Saturation

After sampling, evaporate the solvent. Then the thin layer plate is placed in the chromatographic tank with developing solvent, but is not immersed in the developing solvent. If the acidic component is separated, acetic acid can be added to the tank for saturation, and if the alkaline component is separated, ammonia can be added to the tank for saturation, so as to improve the separation effect.

(4) Development

There are many ways of development, including ascending development (上行展开), descending development (下行展开), near horizontal development (近水平展开), one-dimensional development (单向展开), two-dimensional development (双向展开) and multiple development (多次展开), etc. There are two types of chromatographic tanks: horizontal and vertical. However, the soft plate can only be

developed in a near horizontal way, that is, the angle between the plate and the horizontal is about 15°. During operation, immerse the end of the thin plate absorbed samples into the developing solvent, cover the tank, and ensure that the developing solvent shall not exceed the original spot of the sample. Under the action of capillary, the solvent will develop along the thin layer surface. After the solvent develops to 4/5 of the total length of the thin layer plate, take out the plate, record the solvent front, and dry it. The hard plate can be blow-dried. For the samples with complex composition leading the overlap of some spots, multiple developing can be used, e.g., two dimensional development, one dimensional multiple development, incremental multiple development and step development.

① Two Dimensional Development

Apply the mixed sample at one corner of the square thin-layer plate, and the solvent will be developed along one direction of the thin-layer plate. Take out the thin-layer plate and evaporate the solvent, turn 90° and then conduct the second development along the vertical direction (Figure 2-7). Different solvent systems can be used to separate the complex mixture.

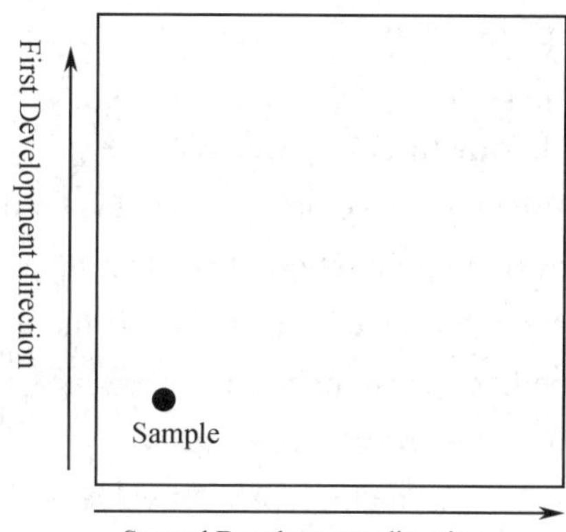

Figure 2-7 Two dimensional development of TLC

② One Dimensional Multiple Development

When the compound can't be separated well after a single development, the developing solvent can be evaporated to dry, and then the plate can be developed at the same distance in the same direction with the same solvent. This operation can be repeated until the separation is satisfactory.

③ Incremental Multiple Development (增量多次展开)

It refers to the repeated development with the same developing solvent in the same direction with incremental distance on the same thin plate. For incremental multiple development, the incremental distance is often the fraction of the length of the thin-layer plate, such as 1/4, 1/2, 3/4, and finally the whole thin-layer length. The incremental multiple developing achieves multiple developments in a short time and provides much better resolution than the general TLC. It is conducive to the concentration of spots and the separation of components with smaller R_f value. Under fixed conditions, the concentrated spots are conducive to improving the separation efficiency and sensitivity.

④ Step Development

When the polarity of the components in the sample differ significantly, it is difficult to separate them on the same thin layer with one developing solution. If two or more different developing solutions are used several times, the components with different polarities can be separated on a thin layer.

(5) Visualization

Some compounds have color, which can be observed under visible light after development. Some compounds will produce fluorescence under the irradiation of UV lamp. After the thin layer is developed, and the solvent evaporates, it can be observed under the UV lamp. Some compounds have no color or fluorescence, so it is necessary to spray the chromogenic reagent to visualize and locate the spots. The soft plate is often blown away by direct spraying of chromogenic reagent. Therefore, it is different from the hard plate in the visualization. The soft plate can be visualized in the following ways.

① **Spraying Method**

When the solvent has not been dried, spray the chromogenic reagent immediately, but do not spray on the surface of the soft plate. Make the chromogenic reagent drop on the plate.

② **Iodine Vapor Method**

Evaporate all the developing solvent after developing. Dry it under the infrared lamp if necessary. Then place it in a sealed tank containing iodine vapor to develop color, many compounds can form brown spots with iodine.

③ **Pressing Plate Method**

After the thin layer is developed, when the developing agent has not evaporated, use another glass plate of the same size with uniform the chromogenic reagent to cover on the thin layer and press to develop color.

④ **Side Sucking Method**

When the developing reagent is completely evaporated after development, one side perpendicular to the developing direction of the thin layer plate is slightly immersed chromogenic reagent to conduct side sucking color development. But if the tested compound can be developed by the chromogenic reagent, this method cannot be used.

(6) Recording the Results

After chromatography, Rf value of the sample was obtained according to the calculation formula.

3.2.3 Precautions

(1) The amount of the sample should not be too much. The diameter of sample spots should not be too large. For sample with large amount, apply the sample for several times with small volume. In addition, the distance between spots should be appropriate. To avoid the influence of edge effect, the sample spots on both sides should have a certain distance from the edge of the thin-layer plate. And what is the most important thing, do not puncture the surface of the thin layer plate.

(2) When developing, the solvent front cannot be expanded to the top or beyond the top of the thin layer plate. Otherwise, the rising height of the solvent cannot be determined, and the R_f value cannot be accurately calculated.

(3) The commonly used adsorbents for TLC are silica gel G [containing 13%–15% gypsum (石膏)], silica gel H (pure silica gel), alumina, etc., which are polar adsorbents. According to the polarity of the separated sample, activation before use is considered. Generally, in order to increase the binding degree between the adsorbent and the separated sample, the water contained in the adsorbent should be removed when separating the compounds with small polarity. In the separation of the components with large polarity, in order to avoid firm adsorption with the adsorbent, a certain amount of water should be properly added to the adsorbent to reduce its adsorption capacity.

重点小结

中药化学成分的提取、分离和检识是中药化学实验的重要操作环节，不仅要理解常用方法的原理，更要掌握基本操作方法。

（1）中药化学成分主要通过溶剂法进行提取，该方法中包括两部分：一是根据中药化学成分的溶解性和酸碱性选择适宜的提取溶剂；二是根据中药材的性质、中药化学成分的稳定性等选择适宜的提取方式。提取溶剂的选择主要依据“相似相溶”的原理。提取方式则分为浸渍、渗漉、煎煮、回流和连续回流提取法，对于热不稳定的化学成分多采用浸渍和渗漉等冷提取方式，溶剂多用极性大、渗透力强的溶剂；对于热稳定的化学成分，为提高提取效率则常采用煎煮、回流和连续回流等热提取方式。此外，中药中的挥发性成分常采用水蒸气蒸馏法进行提取。

（2）中药化学成分的分离纯化可采用结晶法、溶剂沉淀法、pH 梯度萃取法及柱色谱法。结晶法适用于目标化合物在混合物中含量较高时的分离纯化。溶剂沉淀法是通过改变溶剂的极性或 pH 使杂质或目标化合物沉淀析出，该法主要用于中药化学成分的初步分离，按照操作方式可以分为水提醇沉法（水 / 醇法）、醇提水沉法（醇 / 水法）、碱溶酸沉法和酸溶碱沉法。水 / 醇法多用于分离 / 除去中药材水煎液中的大分子水溶性成分，醇 / 水法多用于分离（除去）中药材醇提取液中的脂溶性成分。碱溶酸沉法适用于将酸性成分（如黄酮、蒽醌）与中性、碱性成分分开。酸溶碱沉法则适用于将碱性成分（如生物碱）与中性、酸性成分分开。具有酸、碱性的中药化学成分的进一步分离可采用 pH 梯度萃取法，即将具有酸性或碱性的成分以游离形式溶解于亲脂性有机溶剂中，采用不同 pH 的缓冲溶液进行萃取，从而将酸性不同或碱性不同的成分分开。目前，中药化学中单体化合物的分离主要依赖于柱色谱法。柱色谱法根据其分离原理可分为吸附柱色谱、分配柱色谱、离子交换色谱和排阻色谱。一般而言，中、小极性化合物可以采用以硅胶、氧化铝等为填料的吸附柱色谱分离；极性化合物可以采用以反相 C18 键合相等为填料的分配柱色谱分离；酸性、碱性和两性化合物的分离可以采用以离子交换树脂为填料的离子交换色谱；大分子化合物可以采用以葡聚糖凝胶为填料的排阻色谱；此外，聚酰胺可以与羰基、酚羟基等形成氢键适用于分离黄酮、蒽醌等含有酚羟基的成分；羟丙基葡聚糖凝胶也可用于分离小分子的成分，例如黄酮苷和苷元的分离。吸附柱色谱可以以干柱和湿柱两种方式装填，样品也有干法和湿法两种形式上样；分配柱色谱、离子交换色谱和排阻色谱则均需以湿柱的方式装填。柱色谱分离多采用梯度洗脱的方式，通过收集、合并含有相同成分的流分获得单体化合物。

（3）中药化学成分的检识分为理化检识和薄层检识。理化检识试剂分为通用型试剂和专属性试剂，通用型试剂可使大部分中药化学成分显色，而专属性试剂则针对某一类化学成分或某一种化学基团显色。薄层色谱根据使用的吸附剂（固定相）不同可以分为硅胶薄层色谱、氧化铝薄层色谱、聚酰胺薄膜、反相薄层等。薄层色谱除用于检识中药化学成分外，还可用于筛选柱色谱分离系统、洗脱条件等。

目 标 检 测

题库

思考题

（1）中药化学成分常用的提取方法有哪些？简述溶剂法中溶剂选择的依据。

（2）将某中药的水煎液依次以石油醚、三氯甲烷或乙酸乙酯、正丁醇进行萃取，将分别获得哪几类中药化学成分？

（3）简述结晶法溶剂选择的注意事项。

（4）根据原理不同，柱色谱分为哪几类？

PPT

Chapter 3 Preliminary Test on Chemical Constituents of Chinese Materia Medica

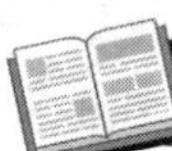
学习目标

知识要求：

1. **掌握** 中药化学成分预实验方法。
2. **熟悉** 主要类型化学成分的常用定性鉴别试剂。
3. **了解** 预实验实例中中药材所含主要化学成分的结构类型。

能力要求：

能够通过系统预实验获知某中药所含化学成分的类型信息。

It is very important to perform the preliminary test before the formal and complete study of chemical constituents of Chinese materia medica. There are two kinds of preliminary test: the single test (单项实验法) (simple and direct examination for searching specific constituents) and the systemic test (系统实验法) (systematic examination for the possible constituents existing in Chinese materia medica without any given information).

Methods of the preliminary test of Chinese materia medica should be simple, fast and accurate. The material can't be directly used in the preliminary test, as the complex interactions among the different constituents. We usually perform the pretreatment (预处理), extract with the solvents with different polarity (from low to high polarity), and finally explore the constituents of different extract to reduce the test range and increase the test accuracy.

1 Purpose and Request

To learn methods and principles of preliminary test on chemical constituents in Chinese materia medica.

To learn how to extract unknown chemical constituents, understand the color or precipitation reaction, master the methods of thin-layer chromatography and paper chromatography, and estimate the categories of constituents according to the results.

2 Preliminary Test Methods

2.1 Sample Preparation

Because different constituents have different solubility in different solvents, we can extract the sample by three kinds of solvents respectively and test them by the following reagents.

2.1.1 Petroleum Ether Extract

Crude powder (1g) is immersed in 10ml petroleum ether (60–90℃) for 2–3h, and then filtered. The filtrate (滤液) is moved to an evaporating dish (蒸发皿) to remove the solvent, and the residue is tested by the following descriptions: Because of possible steroids and triterpenes in the extract, Liebermann-Burchard reaction or 25% phosphomolybdic acid is used; as for possible volatile oils and lipids in the extract, filter paper is usually used to observe if there is oil spot on the paper, and if the spot volatilizes after heating.

2.1.2 Ethanol Extract

Crude powder (10g) is immersed in 5–12 times amount of 95% ethanol, refluxed for 1 hour, and then filtered. Pick up a little of the filtrate directly for the test of phenols (by 1% $FeCl_3$ reagent), tannins [by gelatin (明胶) reagent], and organic acids [by bromothymol blue (溴麝香草酚蓝) reagent]. The remained filtrate is condensed to extract. Some extract is mixed by small amount of 2%–5% HCl, filtered, and the acid liquor is tested for alkaloids by Dragendörff reagent, Mayer reagent, Bertrad reagent, Wagner reagent, or Hager reagent. Some extract is dissolved in a little amount of ethanol for the test of flavonoids (by HCl-Mg reagent or $AlCl_3$) and anthraquinones (by 10% KOH reagent, magnesium acetate reagent or ammonia fumigating). The remained extract is dissolved in a little amount of ethyl acetate, mixed with appropriate amount of 5% NaOH, and moved to a separatory funnel. Phenolic and organic acids should be partitioned in the water layer, and neutral compounds should remain in the organic layer. The ethyl acetate layer is washed to neutral, and evaporated. The obtained residue is dissolved in small amount of ethanol for the test of lactones and coumarins (by open and closed ring reaction, Emerson reagent, Gibb's reagent, or Ferric hydroxamate reagent), and cardiac glycosides (by Kedde reagent, Legal reagent, or Baljet reagent).

2.1.3 Water Extract

Crude powder (10g) is immersed in 100ml water, heated on a water bath at 50–60℃ for 1 hour, and filtered. The filtrate is tested by the following descriptions: as for possible saccharides or glycosides in the extract, Molish reagent or 1% Fehling reagent is used; as for possible organic acids, pH test paper or bromothymol blue reagent is used; as for possible saponins, foam test is performed; as for possible phenolics, 1% $FeCl_3$ reagent is used; as for possible tannins, 1% $FeCl_3$ or gelatin reagent is used; as for possible amino acids, ninhydrin (水合茚三酮) reagent is used; as for possible proteins, biuret (双缩脲) reagent is used; as for possible alkaloids, Dragendörff reagent or Bertrad reagent is used.

2.2 Preliminary Test Methods

In fact, test-tube and filter paper are usually adopted to explore the different kinds of constituents in Chinese materia medica.

2.2.1 Examination of Alkaloids

Alkaloids react with some reagents in acid aqueous solution or diluted ethanol to offer double salt or complex which are hard to dissolve in water. Ammonia dilution is added to the alcohol extract to adjust pH to moderate, and evaporated to dry by water bath. 5% H_2SO_4 solution is then added to dissolve the residue, and filtered. The filtrate is collected for preliminary test.

(1) Mayer Reagent

Mayer reagent (1–2 drops) is added to 1ml filtrate, and alkaloids may exist when pale yellow and white precipitate appeared.

(2) Dragendörff Reagent

Dragendörff reagent (1–2 drops) is added to 1ml filtrate, and alkaloids and compounds containing nitrogen can react with this reagent and yield orange products. Some lactones can also react with this reagent.

(3) Silicotungstic Acid Reagent

Silicotungstic acid reagent (1–2 drops) is added to 1ml filtrate, and alkaloids may exist when pale yellow or grayish-white precipitate appeared.

Note: Alkaloid precipitate reaction needs to occur in acid aqueous solution or acid ethanol dilution because alkaloids and precipitates can be dissolved in such solutions. Meanwhile, trinitrophenol can be reacted under neutral condition. False negative or positive reactions should be noted when using precipitate reaction to estimate alkaloids. Generally secondary amine is hard to react to alkaloid precipitate reagent, such as ephedrine (麻黄碱). Caffeine (咖啡因) does not react with these reagents either. When proteins, polypeptides and tannins exist in solution, such positive reactions could occur also, thus such constituents should be removed from the test solution beforehand. The following processes may be performed to remove such constituents. Basify the acid aqueous solution, extract the solution with chloroform, and separate the chloroform phase, then extract chloroform phase with acid aqueous. Hence, the above interferences are removed from the acid aqueous phase and can be used as testing solution for precipitate reaction. Additionally, all reagents mentioned above should be used respectively to identify alkaloids. Tests are more reliable when all the results are positive or negative.

2.2.2 Examination of Amino Acids, Polypeptides and Proteins

(1) Biuret Reagent

1% $CuSO_4$ solution (1ml) and 1% NaOH solution (1ml) are mixed and added to 1ml cold-water extract, and polypeptides or proteins may exist when violet red appeared after shaking.

(2) Ninhydrin Reagent

0.2% Ninhydrin ethanol solution (2–3 drops) is added to 1ml cold-water extract, shaken, heated on a boiling water bath for 5min, and cooled down. Polypeptides and proteins may exist when blue or amethyst appeared.

2.2.3 Examination of Organic Acids

(1) pH Test Paper

Hot-water and ethanol extracts are determined by pH test paper, and free acids or phenolics may exist when acidity appeared.

(2) Bromothymol Blue Reagent

Ethanol extract is spotted on the filter paper and sprayed with 0.1% bromothymol blue reagent, and organic acids may exist when yellow spot appeared on blue background.

2.2.4 Examination of Phenolics and Tannins

(1) 1% $FeCl_3$ Reagent

1% $FeCl_3$ reagent (1–2 drops) is added to 1ml ethanol extract, and phenolics or tannins may exist when blue greenish-black or amethyst appeared.

(2) Vanillin-Hydrochloride Acid Reagent

Ethanol extract is spotted on the filter paper and vanillin-hydrochloride acid reagent is sprayed after drying, and resorcinol (间苯二酚) compound may exist when different degree of red appeared.

(3) $FeCl_3$-$K_3Fe(CN)_6$ Reagent

Ethanol extract is spotted on the filter paper and $FeCl_3$-$K_3Fe(CN)_6$ reagent is sprayed. Tannins, phenolics and reducing compounds may exist when blue spot appeared. As tannins can react with alkaloids or gel to precipitate, tannins can be removed for the further determination of normal phenolics or tannins.

2.2.5 Examination of Reducing Sugar, Polysaccharides and Glycosides

(1) Fehling Reagent

Fresh Fehling reagent (4–5 drops) is added to 1ml hot-water extract and heated on a water bath for 10min; reducing sugar or other reducing compounds may exist when umber precipitate appeared. To determine polysaccharides and glycosides, 1ml Fehling reagent is added to 4ml water extract, heated on a boiling water bath for 10min, and filtered. The filtrate is acidified by 10% HCl, additional 1ml HCl is added, heated on a boiling water bath for half an hour. Aglycones may exist when suspended matter appeared. After filtration, 10% NaOH and Fehling reagent are added and heated, polysaccharides or glycosides may exist when umber precipitate appeared.

(2) Molish Reagent

5% α-Naphthol ethanol solution (2–3 drops) is added to water and ethanol extracts, shaken well, and small amount of concentrated H_2SO_4 was then added along the test-tube wall. Saccharides, polysaccharides, and glycosides may exist when purple circle appeared on the contact face of H_2SO_4.

(3) Phthalic Acid-Aniline Reagent

Hot-water extract is spotted on the filter paper, and phthalic acid-aniline reagent is sprayed and heated at 105℃ for a few minutes; reducing sugar may exist when brown or brownish red appeared.

2.2.6 Examination of Saponins

(1) Foam Test

Hot-water extract (1–2ml) is added into a test-tube, and shaken thoroughly. If generous honeycomb foam is produced, saponins may exist when the foam does not become less after standing for over 15min or adding ethanol.

(2) Liebermann-Burchard Reaction

Ethanol extract (1–2ml) is evaporated to dry, the residue is dissolved or suspended in acetic anhydride, and then 1 drop sulfuric acid is added. Steroids, triterpenes and saponins may exist when purple appeared and turned to green at upper layer of the solution.

2.2.7 Examination of Steroids and Triterpenes

Liebermann-Burchard reaction is used. 3ml Ethanol extract is evaporated to dry, the residue is dissolved in glacial acetic acid, and 1ml acetic anhydride and 1 drop sulfuric acid are added in turn. Steroid sapogenin, sterol, and triterpenes may exist when the test-tube color gradually changed from yellow to red, purple, blue greenish-black, the color of steroid change faster than triterpenes do.

2.2.8 Examination of Flavonoids

(1) Hydrochloride Acid-Magnesium React

Ethanol extract (1ml) is placed to a test-tube, small amount of magnesium powder is added, then a few drops concentrated hydrochloride acid is added (heated when necessary). Flavonoid may exist when red-purple appeared.

(2) Base Aqueous Assay

Ethanol extract is spotted on the filter paper, and exposed to ammonium vapor. When yellow appeared, flavonoid may exist when the yellow fade after the filter paper leave from ammonium vapor.

(3) Aluminum Trichloride Reagent

The sample is spotted on the filter paper, 1% $AlCl_3$ ethanol reagent is sprayed, and dried. Flavonoids may exist when yellow spot appeared and yellowish-green fluorescence appeared under UV lamp.

2.2.9 Examination of Lactones, Coumarins and Their Glycosides

(1) Fluourescence Assay

Water extract and ethanol extract are spotted on the filter paper, and observed under UV lamp. When blue fluorescence appeared, coumarins and their glycosides may exist when the blue fluorescence turns to yellow after adding base.

(2) Diazotization (重氮化) Assay

3% Na_2CO_3 solution (1ml) is added to 1ml ethanol extract, heated on a water bath to boil for 3min, cooled down, and 1–2 drops fresh diazotization reagent is then added. Coumarins and their glycosides may exist when red appeared.

(3) Ferric Hydroxamic Acid Assay

Hydroxylamine hydrochloride (5 drops) in saturated ethanol and 10 drops NaOH in saturated ethanol are added to ethanol extract, heated to appearance of bubble, cooled down, acidified by 5% hydrochloride, and 1% $FeCl_3$ solution is then added. Ester, lactones, coumarins and their glycosides may exist when pink or purple appeared.

2.2.10 Examination of Cardiac Glycosides

(1) Kedde Reagent

Kedde reagent (4–5 drops) is added to 0.5ml ethanol extract, and cardenolide glycoside may exist when red or purple appeared.

(2) Baljet Reagent

Baljet reagent (1 drop) is added to 1ml ethanol extract, and cardenolide glycoside may exist when orange or red appeared.

(3) Legal Reagent

Ethanol extract (1ml) is evaporated on a water bath to dry, the residue is dissolved with 1ml pyridine, 4–5 drops 0.3% natrium nitroferrocyanatum reagent is added, shaken well, 1–2 drops 10% NaOH solution is then added and shaken well; cardenolide glycoside may exist when red appeared and then fades gradually.

2.2.11 Examination of Anthraquinones

(1) 1% Boric Acid Aqueous Solution

Ethanol extract is spotted on the filter paper, and 1% boric acid aqueous solution is sprayed. Anthraquinones and its glycosides may exist when orange, red or fluorescence appeared.

(2) 5% KOH Aqueous Solution

Ethanol extract is spotted on the filter paper, and 5% KOH aqueous solution is sprayed. Anthraquinones and its glycosides may exist when orange, red, or fluorescence appeared.

(3) Alkali Assay

1% NaOH (1ml) is added to 1ml ethanol extract, small amount of 30% H_2O_2 is added when red appeared, and heated. After acidifying with acidic aqueous solution, the fade of red color indicates the existence of anthraquinone and its glycoside.

2.2.12 Examination of Volatile Oils

The existence of volatile oil can be indicated by the flavor of water extract. Ethanol extract is spotted on the filter paper, essential oil may exist when the oil spot volatilizes naturally.

3 Examples of Preliminary Test

3.1 Preparation of Sample Solution

The powders of the following five Chinese materia medica (0.5g) are immersed in 5ml 95% ethanol respectively, heated on a water bath for 15min, filtered, and the filtrates are taken for the examination of different constituents.

3.2 Methods for Preliminary Test

3.2.1 Examination of Alkaloids

Precipitation react (Dragendörff reagent) is used for examination. Extract of *Stephania tetrandra* S. Moore (粉防己) (0.5ml) is moved on porcelain (瓷) board, 1–2 drops Dragendörff reagent is added, and alkaloids may exist when red appeared.

3.2.2 Examination of Anthraquinones

Bornträger reaction (react with lye) is used for examination. Extract of *Polygonum cuspidatum* Sieb. et Zucc (虎杖) (0.5ml) is moved on porcelain board, 1–2 drops 2% NaOH solution is added, and anthraquinones and their glycosides may exist when red appeared.

3.2.3 Examination of Flavonoids

Hydrochloric acid magnesium reaction is used for examination. Extract of *Sophora japonica* (槐) (0.5ml) is moved on porcelain board, 0.5mg magnesium powder is added, and 5 drops concentrated hydrochloric acid is then added. Flavonoids may exist when red-purple appeared.

3.2.4 Examination of Coumarins

Fluorescence reaction is used for examination. Extract of *Psoralea corylifolia* (补骨脂) is spotted on the filter paper, and observed under UV lamp (365nm). Coumarins may exist when the blue fluorescence turns to yellow after adding base, and fluorescence intensity increases.

3.2.5 Examination of Steroids, Triterpenes, and Their Glycosides

Liebermann-Burchard reaction is used for examination. Extract of glycyrrhizin (2ml) is moved to a test-tube, evaporate on a water bath, 0.5ml acetic anhydride is added to dissolve the residue, and then 0.5ml sulfuric acid is added slowly along the test-tube wall. Red appears at the contact face of acetic anhydride and sulfuric acid, and the color turns purple-blue-green (or yellow-red-purple-blue greenish black) gradually. It indicates the existence of steroids, triterpenes and their glycosides. The phenomenon of steroids and triterpenes is different. The speed of color change of steroids is faster than that of triterpenes.

重点小结

通过预实验可以对中药材中的化学成分类型有初步的了解，从而设计有针对性的提取、分离和检识方法开展中药化学成分研究。一般可将药材用不同溶剂，如石油醚、乙醇、水提取，分别获得石油醚提取液（主要可能含有油脂、蜡、叶绿素、挥发油、游离甾体及三萜类化合物），乙醇提取液（主要可能含有生物碱及其盐、有机酸、黄酮和香豆素的苷及苷元、鞣质等极性化合物），水提取液（主要含有氨基酸、糖类、无机盐等水溶性成分）。随后再采用专属性试剂鉴定各提取液中的化合物种类，为进一步设计提取、分离方法奠定基础。

目标检测

题库

思考题

（1）某中药材的预实验结果如下：石油醚提取物可发生 Liebermann-Burchard 反应、与溴麝香草酚蓝、三氯化铁试剂显色。乙醇提取物可发生 Molish 反应和 HCl-Mg 反应，此外还能与碘化铋钾、硅钨酸和苦味酸生成沉淀。水提取物可发生 Molish 反应，此外还可与雷氏铵盐生成沉淀。试推断其含有哪些类型的化学成分？

（2）设计一个预实验分析中药山楂中含有哪些类型的化学成分。

Chapter 4 Representative Experiments for Extraction, Isolation and Identification of Chemical Constituents from Chinese Materia Medica

PPT

1 Anthraquinones（蒽醌类）

Anthraquinones are oxidized anthracene (蒽) nucleus with carbonyl at position-9 and 10. The phenolic or enolic hydroxyl groups, as well as carboxyl group on anthraquinones, contribute to the acidity of them. So the extraction and isolation methods are always designed according to their acidity. In this section, Polygoni Cuspidati Rhizoma et Radix (虎杖) and Rhei Radix et Rhizoma (大黄) are taken as representative materials for introduction to the extraction, isolation and identification methods of anthraquinones.

1.1 Extraction, Isolation and Identification of Anthraquinones and Polydatin from Polygoni Cuspidati Rhizoma et Radix

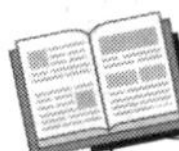

学习目标

知识要求：

1. **掌握** 用pH梯度萃取法分离酸性不同的游离蒽醌的原理及实验方法。
2. **熟悉** 脂溶性成分（苷元）和水溶性成分（苷）的分离方法。
3. **了解** 蒽醌类成分的一般性质和检识反应。

能力要求：

学会采用pH梯度萃取法分离中药中的酸性成分，以及采用柱色谱（硅胶、氧化铝）纯化中药化学成分的方法。

1.1.1 Introduction

Polygoni Cuspidati Rhizoma et Radix is the dried rhizome and root of *Polygonum cuspidatum* Sieb. et Zucc. Its flavor is slightly bitter and property is lightly cold. It enters the liver, gallbladder and lung channels. It has effects of dissolving dampness to eliminate jaundice, reducing heat in blood and counteract toxicity, eliminating stasis to stop pain, stopping cough and dissolving phlegm. It can be used

in treatment of jaundice caused by dampness-heat, turbid flow, rheumatic arthritis, burns, and cough caused by lung-heat, etc. Anthraquinones and stilbenes (二苯乙烯类) are abundant in it. The content of emodin, a free form anthraquinone, should not be less than 1.6%. The content of polydatin, a stibene glycoside, should be not less than 0.15%.

1.1.2 Principles

(1) Structures and Physicochemical Properties of Major Constituents

① **Chrysophanol (大黄酚)**

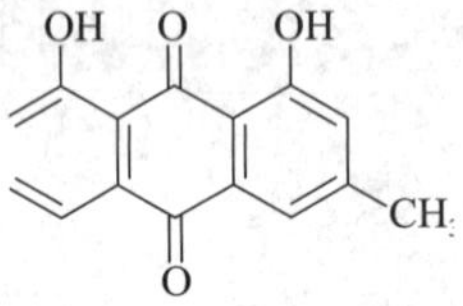

Its melting point is 196℃ and it can sublimate. It is yellow crystals when it is crystallized from acetone and it is needle crystals from ethanol. It can easily dissolve in benzene, chloroform, ethyl ether, NaOH aqueous solution, and hot water, but slightly dissolve in methanol, and hardly dissolve in petroleum ether and cold Na_2CO_3 or $NaHCO_3$ aqueous solution.

② **Emodin (大黄素)**

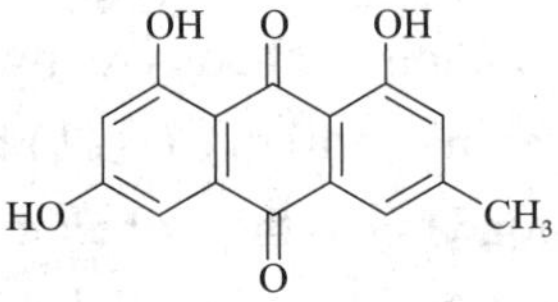

Its melting point is 256–257℃ and it can sublimate. It is orange yellow crystals when it is crystallized from acetone and it is yellow crystals from methanol. Its solubility (w/v) is: 0.14% in Et_2O, 0.01% in CCl_4, 0.07718% in $CHCl_3$. It can easily dissolve in ethanol, and can dissolve in ammonia aqueous, Na_2CO_3 aqueous solution, but hardly dissolved in water.

③ **Physion (大黄素甲醚)**

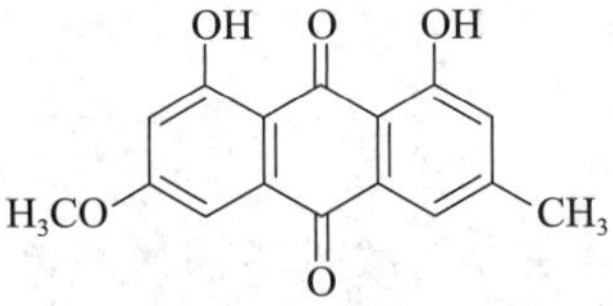

Its melting point is 207℃ and it can sublimate. It is orange yellow needle crystals and its solubility is similar to that of chrysophanol.

④ **Physion-8-*O*-*β*-D-glucoside (大黄素甲醚 -8-*O*-*β*-D- 葡萄糖苷)**

Its melting point is 230–232℃. It is yellow needle crystals when it is crystallized from methanol.

⑤ **Emodin-3-*O*-*β*-D-glucoside (大黄素 -3-*O*-*β*-D- 葡萄糖苷)**

Its melting point is 190–191℃. It is light yellow needle crystals when it is crystallized from ethanol.

⑥ **Polydatin (虎杖苷)**

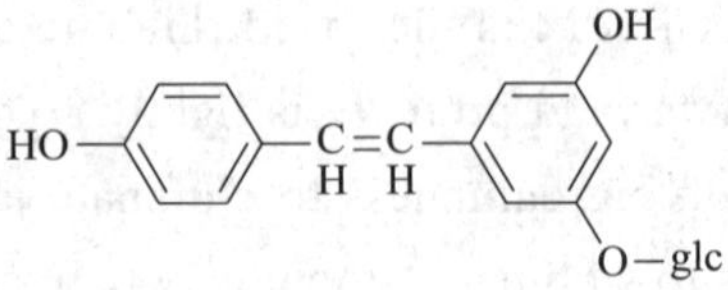

The other name of polydatin is 3, 4', 5-trihydroxystilbene-3-*O*-β-D-glucoside. Its melting point is about 225℃ and it is decomposed at 232℃. It is colorless needle cluster crystals and can be easily dissolved in methanol, ethanol, acetone and hot water. It can also dissolve in ethyl acetate, but slightly dissolve in Na_2CO_3 aqueous solution, and not dissolve in ethyl ether.

UV: λ_{max} (MeOH) nm (log ε) 216 (4.42), 230 sh (4.29), 303(4.52), 318(4.52).

IR: υ_{KBr} (cm^{-1}) 3400, 1600, 1525, 1470, 1270, 1185, 1160, 1100, 1040, 970, 850, 690.

⑦ **Resveratrol (白藜芦醇)**

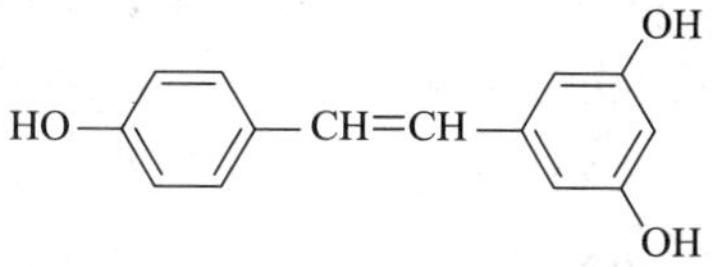

It is colorless needle crystals. Its melting points are at 256–257℃ and 261–264℃. It can sublimate. It can easily dissolve in ethyl ether, chloroform, methanol, ethanol, acetone, etc.

(2) Pharmacological Activities

Anthraquinones from Polygoni Cuspidati Rhizoma et Radix has effects of anti-inflammatory, antisepsis, purgative, diuresis, antitumor, antivirus. It can be used for treatment of hyperlipemia, burns, scald and so on.

Stilbenes from Polygoni Cuspidati Rhizoma et Radix has effects of antioxidation, blood lipids regulating, antitumor, cardiovascular protecting, anti-bacteria, and anti-fungus, etc.

(3) Principle of Extraction and Separation

① Lipophilic constituents (free anthraquinones) and hydrophilic constituents (glycosides) in Polygoni Cuspidati Rhizoma et Radix can be separated by using different organic solvents in partition. According to the difference of solubility between free anthraquinones and glycosides, free anthraquinones can be extracted by ethyl ether or the mixture of cyclohexane and ethyl acetate, and then they are separated from glycosides.

② Free anthraquinones have different acidities due to the different numbers and positions of hydroxyl groups in their structures. Therefore, different alkaline aqueous (5% $NaHCO_3$, 5% Na_2CO_3, 2% NaOH) can extract different acidic constituents from the ethyl ether or the mixture of cyclohexane and ethyl acetate layer. This technique is called pH gradient partition.

1.1.3 Materials and Reagents

Plant material: Crude powder of Polygoni Cuspidati Rhizoma et Radix, 50g.

Reference substances: Emodin, physion, polydatin.

Reagents: $NaHCO_3$, Na_2CO_3, NaOH, Al_2O_3 (100–200 mesh), pH test paper, hydrochloric acid, 85%–95% ethanol, 80% ethanol, cyclohexane, ethyl acetate, $CHCl_3$, MeOH, 0.5% $Mg(Ac)_2$ solution.

Development solvent systems:

A. Petroleum ether (b.p. 30–60℃) -ethyl formate-formic acid (15 : 5 : 1, upper layer).

B. $CHCl_3$-MeOH (9 : 2).

Visualization: 5%KOH/MeOH; 1% $FeCl_3$-1% $K_3[Fe(CN)_6]$ solution (1 : 1, mix before use).

1.1.4 Methods

(1) Extraction

Crude powder of Polygoni Cuspidati Rhizoma et Radix 50g are refluxed with 85%–95% ethanol twice (200ml, 1h; 150ml, 30min), filtered with cotton, combined the filtrate together and concentrated to small volume (about 30ml), then transfer to evaporating dish to evaporate until no alcohol smell. The residue will be the total extract of Polygoni Cuspidati Rhizoma et Radix. Use about 40ml water to suspend, and transfer the total extract to a 100ml flask.

(2) Isolation

① Separation of Free Anthraquinones from Glycosides

Transfer the above aqueous of total extract from Polygoni Cuspidati Rhizoma et Radix into a 500ml separatory funnel, extract 6 times (30ml × 2, 25ml × 4) with the mixture (1 : 3) of cyclohexane and ethyl acetate, combine the organic layers together to yield the solution of total free anthraquinones. Keep for next process. The aqueous layer containing polydatin should be transferred to a flask to keep for the isolation of polydatin.

② Isolation of Free Anthraquinones

a. Isolation of Emodin

Transfer the organic layer solution containing total free anthraquinones to a 500ml separatory funnel, extract 4 times (20ml × 2, 15ml × 2) with 5% $NaHCO_3$ aqueous solution, discharge the 5% $NaHCO_3$ solution; Then the organic layer is extracted 7 times (25ml × 2, 20ml × 5) with 5%Na_2CO_3 aqueous solution. Combine the aqueous layers together and evaporate on water bath to remove the left organic solvents in aqueous solution, cool to room temperature. Drop 6mmol/L HCl to pH 2 with stirring, stand for a moment, filter in vacuum, wash the precipitate to neutral with water, dry, weigh. Then it will be the crude emodin. The organic layer should keep for the isolation of physion.

Dissolve the crude emodin with 20ml cyclohexane-acetone (7 : 3), subject to silica gel column chromatography (100–200 meshes, 15g, ϕ = 2cm), elute with cyclohexane-acetone (7 : 3) at 4–5ml/min speed. Collect the eluate till the orange band being eluted. Concentrate the eluate to dry, and the residue is dissolved with about 5ml ethanol and transferred to a little flask. That will be the solution of emodin, stand for crystallization.

b. Isolation of Physion

The organic layer extracted by 5% Na_2CO_3 aqueous is followed by extracting with 2% NaOH aqueous 5 times (10ml × 5), combine the aqueous layers together and evaporate on water bath to remove the left organic solvents in aqueous solution, cool to room temperature. Drop 6mmol/L HCl to pH 2 with stirring, stand for a moment, filter in vacuum, wash the precipitate to neutral with water, dry, weigh. Then it will be the crude physion.

c. Isolation of Polydatin

The water layer remained in "① The separation of free anthraquinones from glycosides" is transferred to beaker and dilute with water to 150ml. Stir, then filter to remove insoluble impurity. Transfer the filtrate to a 500ml separatory funnel, extract with ethyl acetate for 6 times (40ml × 3, 30ml × 3), combine the ethyl acetate layers together and concentrate to dry. Dissolve the residue with 80% ethanol and subject to Al_2O_3 column (neutral Al_2O_3, 100–200 meshes, diameter is about 2cm, packing the column by the drying method), elute with 80% ethanol (about 100ml), collect the eluate (be aware of not eluting out the red band) and concentrate to dry. Dissolve the residue with 85% EtOH, transfer to a small flask, keep for crystallization, then it will be polydatin.

(3) Identification

① TLC Identification

a. TLC of Free Anthraquinones

Adsorbent: Silica gel TLC plate.

Reference substances: Emodin and physion (1mg/ml ethanol solution,1μl).

Test solution: Self-isolated emodin and physion in ethanol (2μl).

Development solvent system: Petroleum ether (30–60℃) - ethyl formate - formic acid (15 : 5 : 1, upper layer).

Visualization: A. Observing fluorescence under UV lamp at 365nm.

B. Spraying 5% KOH/MeOH solution.

b. TLC of Polydatin

Adsorbent: Silica gel TLC plate.

Reference substance: The ethanol solution of polydatin (1g/ml,1μl).

Test solution: Self-isolated polydatin in ethanol (2μl).

Development solvent system: $CHCl_3$-MeOH (9 : 2).

Visualization: A. Observing fluorescence under UV lamp at 365nm.

B. Spraying 1% $FeCl_3$-1% $K_3[Fe(CN)_6]$ solution (1 : 1 mix before use).

② Color Reactions for Free Anthraquinones

To perform reactions below using ethanol solutions of emodin and physion as test solutions:

Bornträger reaction: 1ml test solution, dropwise 2% NaOH solution, observing the color of solutions.

$Mg(Ac)_2$ reaction: 1ml test solution, dropwise 0.5% $Mg(Ac)_2$ solution, observing the color of solutions.

1.1.5 Procedure Scheme (Figure 4-1)

1.1.6 Precautions

(1) Before the concentrated extract is suspended in water, ethanol should be completely evaporated to no smell of alcohol.

(2) In the isolation of free anthraquinones, don't shake thoroughly after adding the alkaline solution (5% Na_2CO_3) in the first two extractions to avoid emulsification (乳化).

重点小结

虎杖是蓼科植物虎杖的干燥根茎和根。虎杖中含有大量的蒽醌类和二苯乙烯苷类成分。这些成分均能溶于乙醇，因此采用乙醇进行回流提取。

根据游离蒽醌与苷类溶解性能的差异，先用乙醚或环己烷-乙酸乙酯（1 : 3）的混合溶剂萃取出游离蒽醌等脂溶性成分，从而使脂溶性成分（游离蒽醌）和水溶性成分（苷类）得到分离。

根据虎杖中游离蒽醌结构中酚羟基数目和位置的不同而具有不同强度的酸性，用碱性强度递增的水溶液（5% $NaHCO_3$，5% Na_2CO_3，2% NaOH）自有机溶剂中分别萃取出不同酸性强弱的游离蒽醌类成分（pH 梯度萃取法），达到分离的目的。

本实验可以分为四次（提取、游离蒽醌与苷的分离；游离蒽醌的分离纯化；虎杖苷的分离纯化；检识）完成。

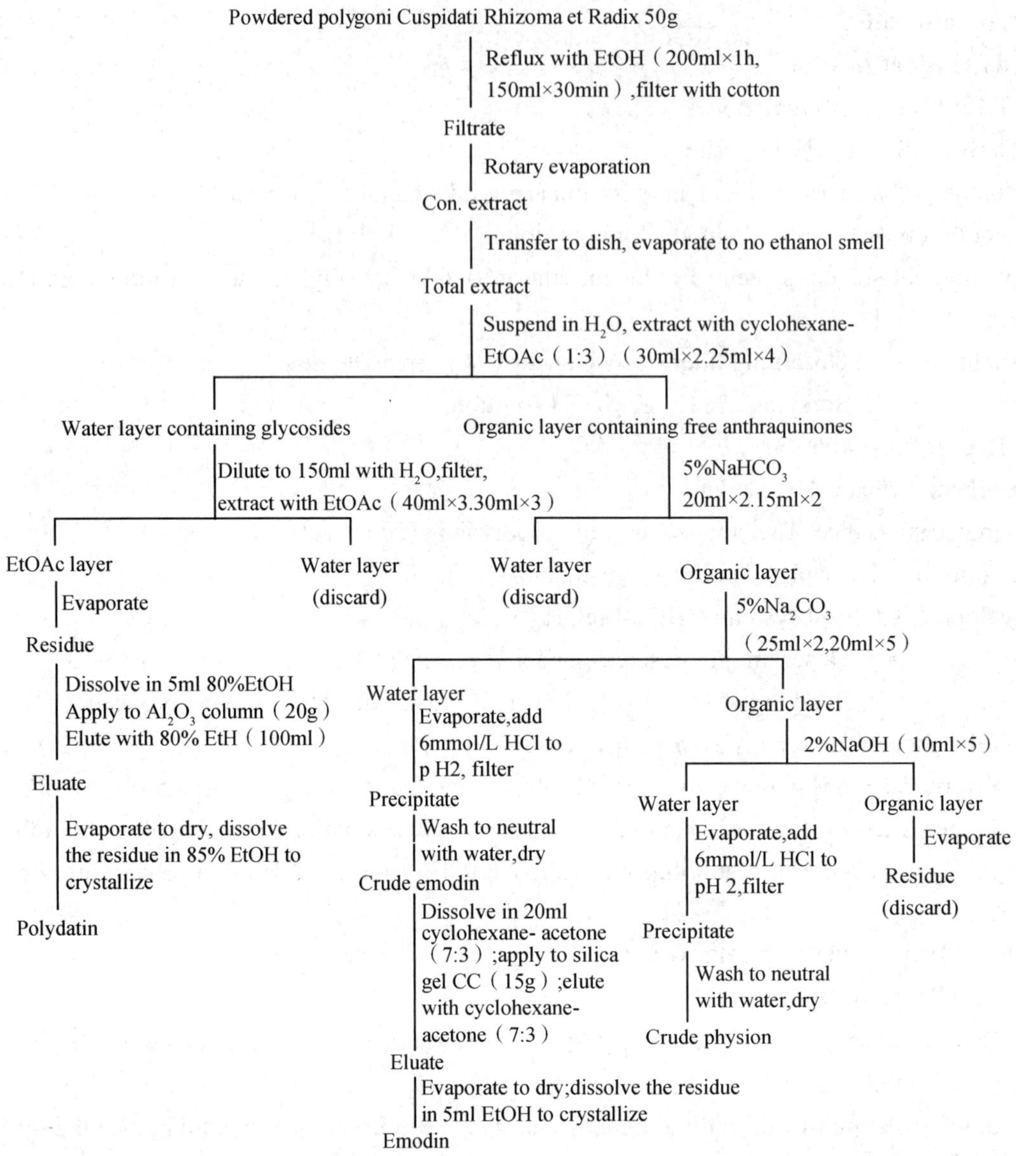

- Powdered polygoni Cuspidati Rhizoma et Radix 50g
  - Reflux with EtOH（200ml×1h, 150ml×30min）,filter with cotton
- Filtrate
  - Rotary evaporation
- Con. extract
  - Transfer to dish, evaporate to no ethanol smell
- Total extract
  - Suspend in H_2O, extract with cyclohexane-EtOAc（1:3）（30ml×2.25ml×4）
  - Water layer containing glycosides
    - Dilute to 150ml with H_2O,filter, extract with EtOAc（40ml×3.30ml×3）
    - EtOAc layer
      - Evaporate
      - Residue
        - Dissolve in 5ml 80%EtOH; Apply to Al_2O_3 column（20g）; Elute with 80% EtH（100ml）
      - Eluate
        - Evaporate to dry, dissolve the residue in 85% EtOH to crystallize
      - Polydatin
    - Water layer (discard)
  - Organic layer containing free anthraquinones
    - 5%$NaHCO_3$ 20ml×2.15ml×2
    - Water layer (discard)
    - Organic layer
      - 5%Na_2CO_3（25ml×2,20ml×5）
      - Water layer
        - Evaporate,add 6mmol/L HCl to p H2, filter
        - Precipitate
          - Wash to neutral with water,dry
        - Crude emodin
          - Dissolve in 20ml cyclohexane- acetone（7:3）;apply to silica gel CC（15g）;elute with cyclohexane-acetone（7:3）
        - Eluate
          - Evaporate to dry;dissolve the residue in 5ml EtOH to crystallize
        - Emodin
      - Organic layer
        - 2%NaOH（10ml×5）
        - Water layer
          - Evaporate,add 6mmol/L HCl to pH 2,filter
          - Precipitate
            - Wash to neutral with water,dry
          - Crude physion
        - Organic layer
          - Evaporate
          - Residue (discard)

Figure 4-1 Extraction and isolation of anthraquinones and polydatin from Polygoni Cuspidati Rhizoma et Radix

目 标 检 测

思考题

（1）简述虎杖中游离蒽醌类成分的分离原理。

（2）根据薄层色谱结果分析大黄素、大黄酚的结构与 R_f 值的关系。

（3）为什么总提物在加水分散前要先浓缩并蒸发到无醇味？

（4）总结萃取操作程序及注意事项。

1.2 Extraction, Isolation and Identification of Anthraquinones from Rhei Radix et Rhizoma

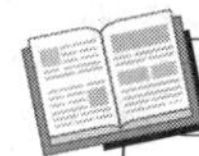

学习目标

知识要求：

1. **掌握** pH梯度萃取法的原理和硅胶柱色谱法的原理。
2. **熟悉** 蒽醌类化合物的检识方法。
3. **了解** 中药大黄的药材基源及药用部位。

能力要求：

学会采用pH梯度萃取法分离中药中的酸性成分，学会采用硅胶柱色谱法分离纯化中药中的化学成分。

1.2.1 Introduction

The roots and rhizomes of *Rheum palmatum* L. (掌叶大黄), *R. offcinale* Baill. (药用大黄), and *R. tanguticum* Maxim.ex Balf. (唐古特大黄) are the sources of Rhei Radix et Rhizoma (大黄), which is widely used to purge heat and remove toxins in Chinese medicine. Modern research indicated that the main effective constituents are anthraquinones and their glycosides. The typical constituents are listed in Table 4-1. Most anthraquinone compounds exist as glycosides, and dianthrones can also be found in the fresh rhubarbs. Sennoside (番泻苷) A, B, C, D are the glycosides of dianthrones.

	R_1	R_2
chrysophanol	CH_3	H
emodin	CH_3	OH
physcion	CH_3	OCH_3
aloe-emodin (芦荟大黄素)	H	CH_2OH
rhein (大黄酸)	H	COOH

Table 4-1 Properties of main anthraquinones in Rhei Radix et Rhizoma

Compound	Crystal form	Solubility
Rhein	Brown needle	Soluble in pyridine, $NaHCO_3$, Na_2CO_3 and NaOH water solution; slightly soluble in ethanol, benzene, ethyl ether, and petroleum ether; insoluble in water
Emodin	Orange needle	Soluble in aqueous solutions of ammonium hydroxide, Na_2CO_3 and NaOH, as well as in ethanol, methanol, acetone, ethyl ether, chloroform; insoluble in water
Chrysophanol	Orange-yellow rectangle or monoclinic	Easily dissolve in aqueous solutions of NaOH and hot ethanol; soluble in benzene, chloroform, ethyl ether, glacial acetic acid, acetone; slightly dissolve in cooled ethanol; insoluble in water
Physcion	Golden-yellow needle	Soluble in benzene, pyridine, chloroform, aqueous solutions of NaOH; slightly dissolve in ethyl acetate, methanol, ethyl ether; insoluble in water and Na_2CO_3 water solution
Aloe-emodin	Orange needle	Easily dissolve in dilute NaOH solution, hot ethanol, acetone, methanol; soluble in pyridine; slightly dissolve in ethanol, benzene, chloroform, ethyl ether and petroleum ether

	R	C_{10}-C_{10}' configuration
Sennoside A	COOH	*trans*
Sennoside B	COOH	*cis*
Sennoside C	CH_2OH	*trans*
Sennoside D	CH_2OH	*cis*

1.2.2 Principles

All the compounds listed above show definite acidity for the presence of phenolic hydroxyl and carboxyl groups in their structure. Due to the different acidity, rhein, emodin, aloe-emodin, physcion, and chyrsophanol can dissolve in alkaline water with different pH values. Figure 4-2 shows the results of the PC with different pH buffer zone, the values of K and β can be calculated. Thus rhein, emodin, and aloe-emodin can be isolated successively by the method of pH gradient partition. The order of acidity of these five compounds is as follows:

Rhein > emodin > aloe-emodin > physcion ≈ chrysophanol

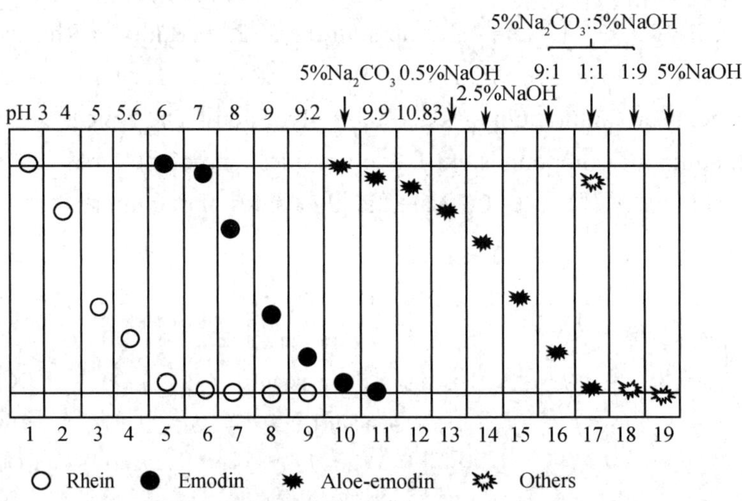

Figure 4-2 Buffer PC of emodin type anthraquinones

1.2.3 Material and Reagents

Material: Rhei Radix et Rhizoma 50g.

Reference substances: rhein, emodin, chyrsophanol.

Reagents: 95% ethanol, diethyl ether, petroleum ether (30–60℃), ethyl acetate, formic acid, acetic acid, chloroform, acetone, cyclohexane, concentrated hydrochloric acid, concentrated sulfuric acid, 5% $NaHCO_3$ solution, 5% Na_2CO_3 solution, 1% NaOH solution, 0.5% $Mg(Ac)_2$ solution, ammonia, pH test paper, silica gel (100–200mesh, 200–300mesh).

1.2.4 Methods

(1) Extraction

Weigh the crude powder of Rhei Radix et Rhizoma 50g in a 500ml round-bottom flask and add 95% ethanol 200ml and reflux for 1h. Then filter and extract the residue again in the same way by 150ml

95% ethanol for 0.5h. Filter and remove the residue. Combine the extractions and remove the ethanol completely in vacuum to get the total extract.

(2) Separation of Free Anthraquinones from Total Extract

Add ethyl ether 50ml to the total extract, immerse for 15min with shaking. Transfer the solution to a 500ml separatory funnel. Then repeat this procedure three times to fully dissolve the free anthraquinones. Thus, the free anthraquinones were in the ethyl ether and the glycosides remain in the residue.

(3) Separation of Rhein, Emodin and Other Free Anthraquinones by pH Gradient Partition

Add 5% $NaHCO_3$ solution 40ml in the separatory funnel. Collect the aqueous layer. Repeat the procedure three times. Combine the aqueous solution in a 250ml beaker and adjust to pH 2 with concentrate hydrochloric acid. Stand still for 10min. Filter in vacuum. Wash the precipitate with a little water till pH of the solution is around neutral. Dry the precipitate to get rhein.

Add 5% Na_2CO_3 solution 40ml in the separatory funnel to extract the ethyl ether layer. Collect the aqueous layer. Repeat the procedure three times. Combine the aqueous solution in a 250ml beaker and adjust to pH 2 with concentrate hydrochloric acid. Stand still for 10min. Filter in vacuum. Wash the precipitate with a little water till pH of the solution is around neutral. Dry the precipitate to get emodin.

Add 2% NaOH solution 40ml in the separatory funnel and extract the ethyl ether layer. Collect the aqueous layer. Repeat the procedure three times. Combine the aqueous solution in a 250ml beaker and adjust to pH 2 with concentrate hydrochloric acid. Stand still for 10min. Filter in vacuum. Wash the precipitate with a little water till pH of the solution is around neutral. Dry the precipitate to get the mixture of aloe-emodin, physcion and chrysophaol.

微课

(4) Separation of Aloe-Emodin, Physcion and Chrysophaol through Silica Gel Column Chromatography

① Selecting Eluting Solvent

a. Selecting Solvent System

Dissolve the mixture in the previous step with suitable solvent and develop silica gel TLC in different solvent systems. Solvent systems of *n*-hexane-EtOAc, petroleum ether-EtOAc, and petroleum ether-acetone are recommended for the isolation of aloe-emodin, physcion and chyrsophanol according to the resolution among spots in the mixture.

b. Selecting Initial Elution

The ratio of the solvents in the suitable system is adjusted to make the R_f of the target spot at 0.2–0.3. The initial elution is applied in the wet column.

② Preparation of Sample

The sample can be prepared in the following two ways.

a. "Dry Sample"

Dissolve the mixture in the previous step with suitable solvent, put the solution into silica gel of 1–3 times weight as much as that of the sample. Stir and let the sample to be adsorbed on the silica gel thoroughly. The solvent is vaporized until no solvent residue.

b. "Wet Sample"

Dissolve the mixture in the previous step in the initial solvent.

③ Column Packing

The amount of the absorbent is 10–30 times weight as much as that of the sample. The column can be packed in the following two ways.

a. Wet Column

Mix silica gel and the initial solvent in a beaker and stir to get uniform slurry without bubbles. Pour the slurry into the column. Open the piston. Let the solvent drop into the collecting bottle. Elute the column bed until the column equilibrates. Let the solvent level down to just above the adsorbent top level.

b. Dry Column

The column is packed with silica gel without solvent. Usually the silica gel with high mesh is used. If necessary, the elution is carried under pressure.

④ Sample Application

a. For "Dry Sample"

Apply the silica gel adsorbing samples on the top of the column.

b. For "Wet Sample"

Drop the sample solution on the top of the column carefully.

⑤ Elution

The general amount of eluting solvent is about 3–5 times of the column volume.

a. For wet column gradient elution is usually used. A gradient solvent system is used by increasing the proportion of the polar solvent.

b. For dry column isometric elution is usually used. The ratio of the elution can also be adjusted based on the actual results of isolation.

⑥ Collection of Fractions

Generally, eluate of 1/10–1/2 of a retention volume is collected as a fraction. After concentrated, the residue is transferred to a sample bottle. Combine the fractions according to TLC detection.

(5) Identification of Anthraquinones from Rhubarb

Dissolve the samples collected from the above procedures, *i.e.* (2) and (3) in 95% EtOH, then use color reaction and TLC to identify the samples.

① Color Reaction

Add 2% NaOH, 0.5% $Mg(Ac)_2$, and concentrated H_2SO_4 to the sample solutions, respectively. Record the color variation of each sample.

② TLC Identification

Adsorbent: Silica gel H-CMC plate.

Reference substances: rhein, emodin, chyrsophanol.

Test solutions: EtOH solutions of the samples.

Development solvent system: Petroleum ether (30–60℃) -ethyl acetate -formic acid (15 : 5 : 1).

Visualization: observe under 365nm UV lamp and then fumigate with ammonia.

1.2.5 Procedure Scheme (Figure 4-3)

1.2.6 Precautions

(1) During the concentration process, the ethanol extract shall be transferred to the flask in several times, and the volume of the solution shall not exceed half of the flask volume. Concentrate until the extract is syrup like, transfer while hot, wash the flask with a small amount of hot ethanol to obtain the total ethanol extract.

(2) When adding ethyl ether to extract the free anthraquinones, do not shake it excessively. Take a clear extract liquid and use it for pH gradient partition. The use of ethyl ether should be operated in hood.

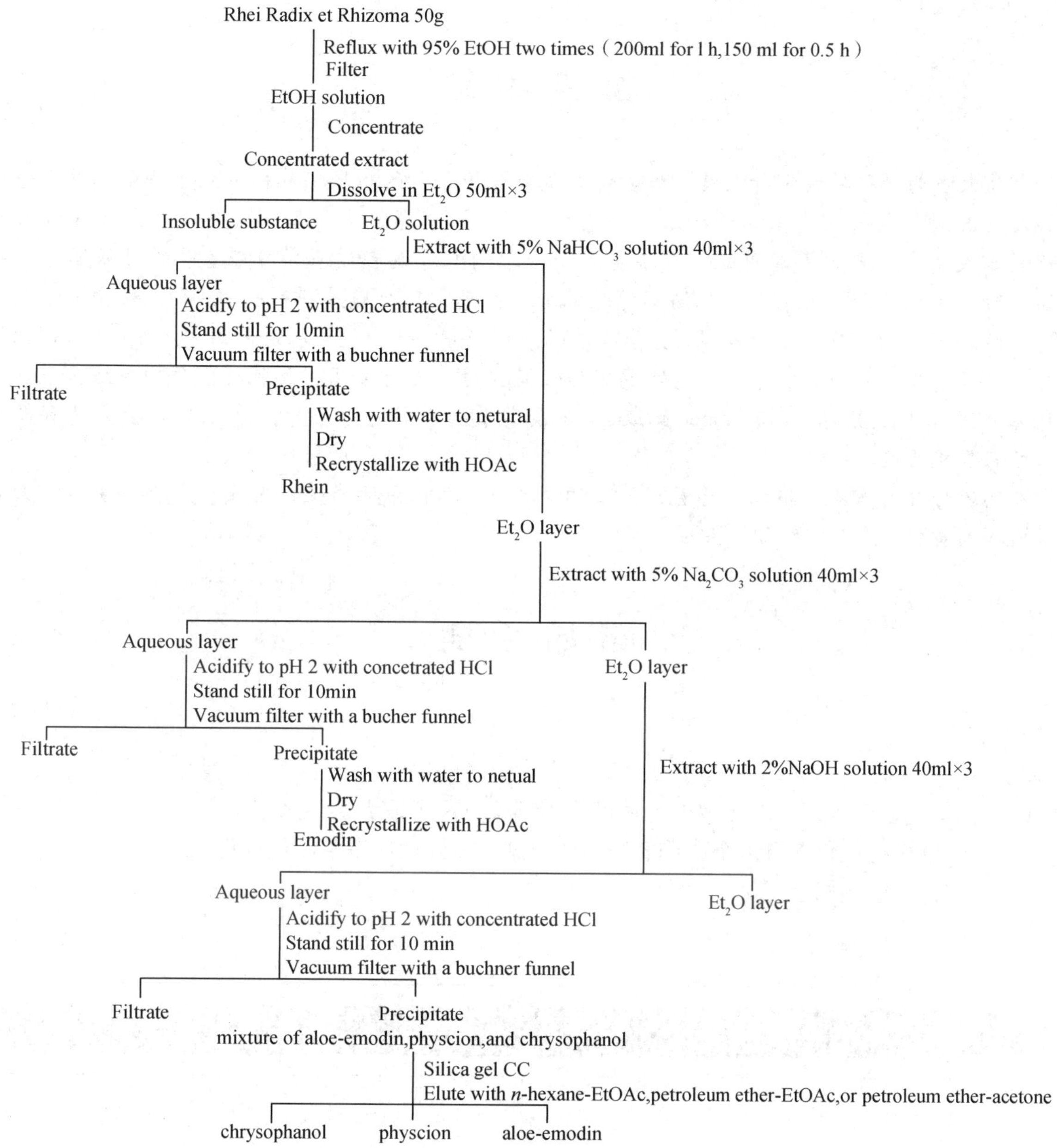

Rhei Radix et Rhizoma 50g

Reflux with 95% EtOH two times (200ml for 1 h, 150 ml for 0.5 h)

Filter

EtOH solution

Concentrate

Concentrated extract

Dissolve in Et_2O 50ml×3

Insoluble substance

Et_2O solution

Extract with 5% $NaHCO_3$ solution 40ml×3

Aqueous layer

Acidify to pH 2 with concentrated HCl

Stand still for 10min

Vacuum filter with a buchner funnel

Filtrate

Precipitate

Wash with water to netural

Dry

Recrystallize with HOAc

Rhein

Et_2O layer

Extract with 5% Na_2CO_3 solution 40ml×3

Aqueous layer

Acidify to pH 2 with concetrated HCl

Stand still for 10min

Vacuum filter with a bucher funnel

Filtrate

Precipitate

Wash with water to netual

Dry

Recrystallize with HOAc

Emodin

Et_2O layer

Extract with 2%NaOH solution 40ml×3

Aqueous layer

Acidify to pH 2 with concentrated HCl

Stand still for 10 min

Vacuum filter with a buchner funnel

Filtrate

Precipitate

mixture of aloe-emodin, physcion, and chrysophanol

Silica gel CC

Elute with *n*-hexane-EtOAc, petroleum ether-EtOAc, or petroleum ether-acetone

chrysophanol

physcion

aloe-emodin

Et_2O layer

Figure 4-3 Extraction and isolation of anthraquinones from Rhei Radix et Rhizoma

(3) A large number of CO_2 bubbles are generated during acidification, so be careful to prevent content overflow.

(4) During the operation of column chromatography, the ratios of the amount of the sample to the weight of the absorbent are usually 1 : 5, 1 : 10, 1 : 30 or 1 : 50. The amount of absorbent should be selected according to the results of TLC. The smaller the resolution between the components in the sample, the greater the amount of absorbent is used. On the contrary, the greater the resolution between the components, the smaller the amount of absorbent is used.

(5) In the process of column packing, if the amount of absorbent is too large and it is difficult to pour it in one time, before pouring it in the second time, use a glass rod to gently stir up the settled silica gel surface poured in the first time, and then pour the remaining silica gel, so as to avoid forming a loose and different layer belt between the two poured silica gel and affect the separation effect.

重点小结

中药大黄为蓼科植物掌叶大黄、唐古特大黄或药用大黄的干燥根和根茎。大黄中主要成分为蒽醌类化合物，包括游离型蒽醌和结合型蒽醌。芦荟大黄素、大黄酸、大黄素、大黄酚和大黄素甲醚是大黄中主要的游离蒽醌。蒽醌类化合物结构中常连有羧基和酚羟基等酸性基团，酚羟基因其所连位置不同酸性有差异。游离蒽醌的酸性强弱按下列顺序排列：$-COOH>2$ 个 $\beta-OH$ > 1 个 $\beta-OH$ >2 个 $\alpha-OH$ >1 个 $\alpha-OH$。依据该性质可采用 pH 梯度萃取法分离大黄中的游离蒽醌。此外，还可依据硅胶对大黄中游离蒽醌的吸附性差异对其进行分离。蒽醌类化合物因结构中含有酚羟基，可与碱液呈色（Bornträger 反应）、与镁离子络合显色，此外，蒽醌中的羰基具有弱碱性，可与强酸呈色。

本实验可分为四次（提取；总游离蒽醌的制备及大黄酸和大黄素的分离；芦荟大黄素、大黄素甲醚和大黄酚的分离；检识）完成。

目标检测

思考题

（1）除采用乙醇加热回流提取外，还可采用哪些方法提取大黄中的化学成分？
（2）经 TLC 检识仍含有多个斑点的样品如何进一步处理获得单体化合物？
（3）蒽醌类化合物还能够发生哪些颜色反应？

2 Flavonoids（黄酮类）

Flavonoids are derivatives of 2-phenylchromone. Most of them have hydroxyl groups contributing the acidity of them. So the extraction and isolation methods are always designed according to their acidity. Besides, due to the hydroxyl groups, polyamide is also used in the isolation and detection of flavonoids. In this section, Sophorae Flos (槐花) is taken as a representative material for introduction to the extraction, isolation and identification methods of flavonoids. As the common method for structure research of glycoside, acidic hydrolyzation is also applied in the identification of flavonoid glycoside from Sophorae Flos.

Extraction, Isolation and Identification of Flavonoids from Sophorae Flos (槐花)

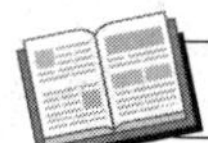

学习目标

知识要求：

1. **掌握** 碱提酸沉法制备芦丁的原理；苷类化合物酸水解的原理；聚酰胺TLC的分离原理；黄酮类和糖类化合物的检识方法。

2. **熟悉** 碱提酸沉法、重结晶、苷类酸水解以及聚酰胺TLC的基本操作。

3. **了解** 中药槐米的药材基源及药用部位；制备液相色谱法在中药化学成分分离中的应用。

能力要求：

学会碱提酸沉法、重结晶、苷类酸水解以及聚酰胺TLC的操作方法；学会黄酮类和糖类化合物的检识方法。

2.1.1 Introduction

The dried flower and flower bud of *Sophora japonica* L. is the source of Soporae Flos (槐花). It is collected in summer at flowering or when flower buds are forming, dried in time and removed from branch, pedicel (花梗) and foreign matters. The flower is known as "Huaihua", and the bud "Huaimi". It is used in hematochezia, hemorrhidal bleeding, dysentery with bloody stools, abnormal uterine bleeding, spitting of blood, epistaxis, bloodshot eyes, headache, and dizziness due to excessive fire in the liver.

It contains high content of rutin (芦丁) (around 23.5%), which is a flavonoid existing in more than 70 kinds of plant. The interesting thing is when the buds bloom, the content of rutin will sharply reduce to 13.0%. In addition to rutin, it also contains betulin (白桦脂醇), sophoradiol (槐二醇), sophorin A (槐花米甲素), sophorins B and C.

Rutin is not only used for the treatment of capillary fragility caused by hemorrhagic disease and hypertension as an adjuvant (辅助药), also as a pharmaceutical material used in the manufacture of quercetin (槲皮素), hydroxyethyl-quercetin, troxerutin (三羟乙基芦丁,曲克芦丁), 2-hydroxypropyl-rutin, β-ethyl morpholine-rutin, 6-diethylamine-methylrutin etc.

Rutin is a flavonoid glycoside. The aglycone is quercetin, and the sugar moiety is rutinose, which is a disaccharide formed by a molecule of glucose and a molecule of rhamnose through 1-6 connection.

HO, O, OH, OH, O, OH, O, O, HO, O, HO, HO, OH, HO, OH, O, OH

2.1.2 Principles

Rutin contains phenolic hydroxyl groups. It can be alkalified to form salt and dissolved in water. When the salt solution is acidified to pH<7, rutin is again in free form and precipitate from water solution. According to this property, rutin is extracted from Soporae Flos and isolated from other kinds of compounds. This method is called alkali extraction and acid precipitation. Rutin can easily dissolve in hot water (1 : 200), but it is insoluble in cold water (1 : 10000). Thus, water is usually applied for the recrystallization of rutin. Rutin is a glycoside. By hydrolysis in acidic condition, rutin degrades to quercetin, glucose and rhamnose.

2.1.3 Material and Reagents

Material: Soporae Flos 30g.

Reference substances: rutin, quercetin, glucose and rhamnose.

Reagents: 95% ethanol, 75% ethanol, concentrated hydrochloric acid, concentrated sulfuric acid, calcium oxide, ammonia, 1% $AlCl_3$ methanol solution, phthalic acid-aniline, magnesium powder, α-naphthol, pH test paper, silica gel TLC plate, polyamide film.

2.1.4 Methods

(1) Extraction of Rutin from Soporae Flos

Place Soporae Flos 30g in a 1000ml beaker, add 300ml water. Under stirring, adjust pH value to 8–9 using lime cream, which is prepared by suspending calcium oxide in water in the ratio of 1 : 10 (w : v). Boil the solution gently for 30min. During this process, maintain the pH value at 8–9 as well as the volume of the water. After boiling, filter the extracted solution with cotton firstly to get rid of the residue, and squeeze the cotton to collect the remaining solution then use a buchner funnel (布氏漏斗) to filter the solution again to get rid of the fine particles. Adjust the pH value to 4–5 with concentrate HCl, stand for at least one night to precipitate rutin, filter in vacuum with buchner funnel and collect the crystals (crude rutin), then dry it in the air.

(2) Purification of Rutin

The purification of rutin can be achieved via recrystallization and prepared HPLC. Half amount of the crude rutin is subjected to purification procedures.

① Purification by Recrystallization

Dissolve the crude rutin in proper amount of water with the approximate ratio at 1 : 200 under heat. Filter the insoluble impurities with a buchner funnel while the solution is hot. Transfer the filtrate in a beaker. After the filtrate cooling down, rutin crystallizes out from the filtrate, then filter and dry the crystal in air or at 60–70℃. Calculate the yield.

② Purification with Prepared HPLC

The crude rutin is dissolved with 55% methanol-water to yield a sample solution with the concentration of 1mg/ml, which is filtered through 0.45μm microporous membrane and injected into the HPLC. The reference chromatographic conditions are as follows.

Column: C_{18} (250mm × 10 mm, 5μm).

Mobile phase: methanol-water (55 : 45).

Flow rate: 3ml/min.

Detection wavelength: 220nm; monitoring wavelength: 360nm.

Injection volume: 1ml.

Under the reference condition, the isolation of each inject can be achieved in approximate 25min, and the retention time of rutin is at about 11min (Figure 4-4).

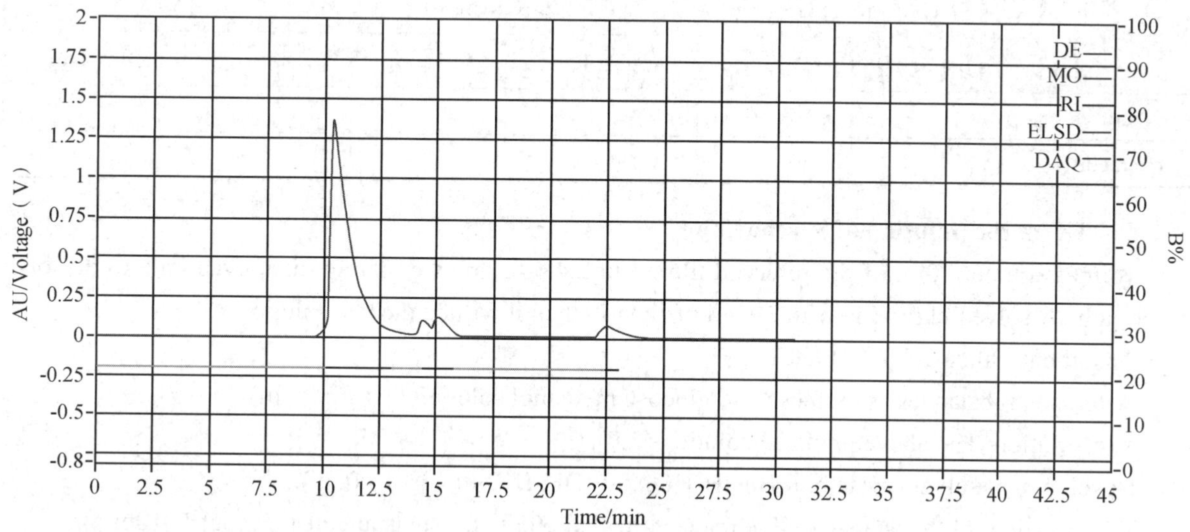

Figure 4-4 Illustration for prepared HPLC of rutin

After several times of injection, the chromatographic peaks are collected in the test tube, and the solvent is removed by vacuum distillation. The residue in the flask is refined rutin.

(3) Acid Hydrolyzation of Rutin

Take the other half amount of crude rutin, add 100ml 1% H_2SO_4, reflux for 1 hour. During this process, the solution will become clear firstly due to the dissolve of rutin, then the solution will be turbid when yellow crystal of quercetin gradually produce. After the hydrolysis, cool down the solution and filter the turbid solution with buchner funnel to get yellow crystal of quercetin after washing with water. Adjust the filtrate (hydrolysate) to neutral with barium carbonate (碳酸钡) powder, then filter to collect the filtrate in a test tube for next step to identify the saccharide generated from the rutin hydrolysis.

(4) Identification of Rutin, Quercetin and the Solution of Saccharide

① Color Reaction of Rutin, Quercetin and Saccharide

Dissolve rutin and quercetin with ethanol. Take proper amount of dissolved solution and conduct the following tests respectively.

HCl-Mg Reaction: Take 1–2ml the solutions of rutin and quercetin, add a little magnesium powder, then add two drops of concentrate HCl, and observe the phenomenon.

Molish Reaction: Take 1–2ml the solutions of rutin, quercetin and saccharide, add a little α-naphthol, shake well, and add concentrate H_2SO_4 of equal volume with sample solution along the tube wall, observe the phenomenon.

② Polyamide Film Chromatography of Rutin and Quercetin

Adsorbent: polyamide TLC plate.

Reference substances: rutin, quercetin.

Test solutions: EtOH solutions of the samples.

Development solvent system: 75% ethanol.

Visualization: Observe under visible light and UV lamp (365nm), respectively. Then put a covered tank saturated with ammonia. After recording the color, wait until the color fades. And finally spray 2% $AlCl_3$ reagent.

Fill the color changes in the following table.

	Hcl-Mg Reaction		Molish Reaction		1%AlCl$_3$	
	visible light	UV lamp	visible light	UV lamp	visible light	UV lamp
rutin						
quercetin						

③ TLC of the Solution of Saccharide

To measure out 20ml of the reserved filtrate in 2.4.3 to an evaporating dish, evaporate to dry on a water bath, dissolve the residue with 2–3ml methanol, then it will be the test solution.

Adsorbent: Silica gel TLC plate.

Reference substances: Rhamnose and glucose methanol solution (1mg/ml, 1μl).

Test solution: The above prepared solution (2μl).

Development solvent system: *n*-BuOH-HOAc-EtOH-H_2O (4 : 1 : 1 : 0.25).

Visualization: Phthalic acid-aniline reagent, heat at 105℃ till spots are clear (about 5–10min).

2.1.5 Procedure scheme (Figure 4-5)

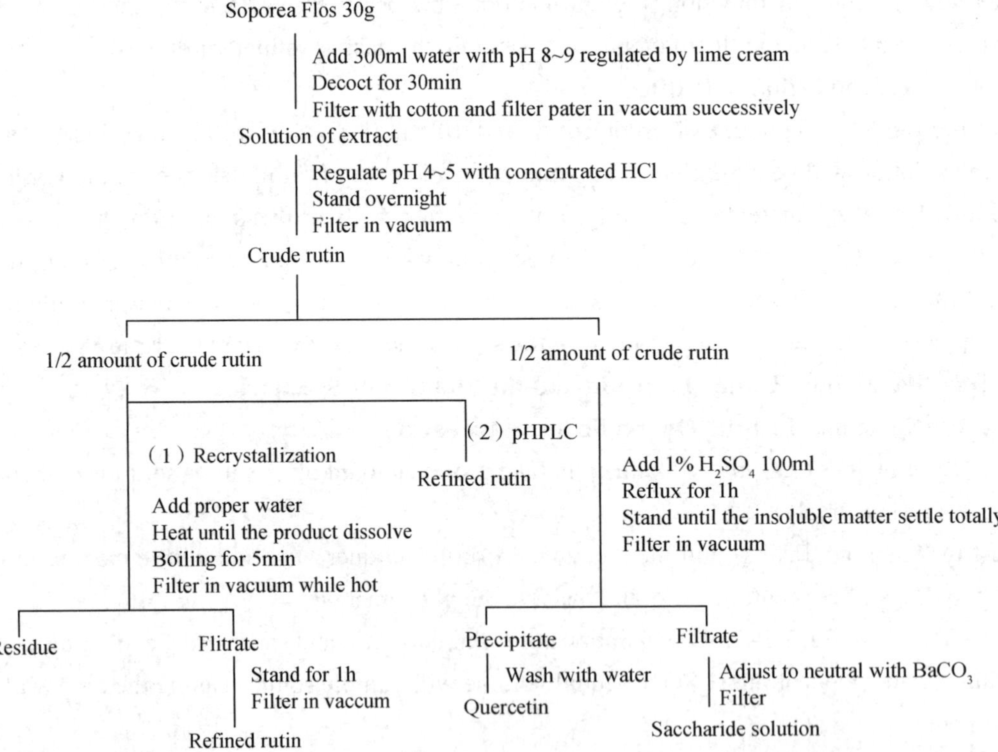

Figure 4-5 Extraction and isolation of flavonoids from Sophorae Flos

2.1.6 Precautions

(1) The evaporation of water leads to the decrease of extraction solvent volume and extraction rate, thus the water volume should be maintained during the boiling process. Adding water and keeping the extracting solution boiling gently are two remedial measures.

(2) To ensure that rutin can be dissolved as salt form, timely supplement the consumed lime cream to maintain the pH value of alkali water.

(3) Adjusting pH value should not exceed the range. The lime cream can not only make rutin become salt, but also remove a large amount of polysaccharide, such as pectin and mucilage contained in Soporae Flos. However, if the pH value is too high, it is easy to destroy the structure of flavonoid nucleus and reduce the yield of rutin. And excessive concentrate hydrochloric acid form oxonium salt with rutin, which will be re-dissolved and the yield of rutin will be reduced.

(4) In the process of recrystallization, the amount of water is in the proportion to the weight of rutin, 15%–20% more than saturation.

(5) In the process of filtration while hot, do not drain in the process of filtration to prevent crystallization on the glass rod. After filtration, transfer the filtrate from the filter flask to the beaker quickly, and let it stand for crystallization.

(6) In Molish reaction, concentrate sulfuric acid should be added along the tube wall without shake to prevent damaging the liquid surface. The height of the two layers of solution should be equal.

重点小结

中药槐花为豆科植物槐的花和花蕾。槐花中主要成分为黄酮类化合物，芦丁是黄酮醇苷，是含量最高的主要指标性成分。芦丁等黄酮类化合物因结构中有酚羟基，具有酸性，可采用碱提酸沉法进行提取，在提取过程中注意调节提取液 pH 至碱性时，加碱不宜过量，否则会破坏黄酮的母核；在提取完毕加酸回调 pH 时，也不宜过量，否则会与黄酮形成鎓盐重新溶解，降低收率。常用的碱液为石灰乳，即氢氧化钙，其既可以使芦丁成盐溶解，也可与药材中的果胶、黏液质等含羧基的杂质形成沉淀，从而达到提取、除杂的双重目的。

芦丁为槲皮素的芸香糖苷（该糖为葡萄糖和鼠李糖连接而成的双糖），其在酸性条件下能够水解生成苷元槲皮素和葡萄糖、鼠李糖。

芦丁及其苷元槲皮素均可发生盐酸－镁粉反应，此外芦丁作为苷还可发生 Molish 反应。

本实验可分为四次（碱提酸沉；芦丁的精制；芦丁的酸水解；检识）完成。

目标检测

思考题

（1）除碱提酸沉法外，还可以采用哪些方法提取黄酮类化合物？

（2）除了结晶法外，还有哪些利用物质的溶解度差异进行分离的操作？

（3）芦丁酸水解过程中水解液由浑浊变澄清、复又浑浊的原因是什么？

3 Coumarins（香豆素）

Coumarins are derivatives of lactones of *o*-hydroxycinnamic acid. So the extraction and identification methods are always designed according to the property of lactone. In this section, Psoraleae Fructus (补骨脂) is taken as a representative material for introduction to the extraction, isolation and identification methods of coumarins.

Extraction, Isolation and Identification of Coumarins from Psoraleae Fructus

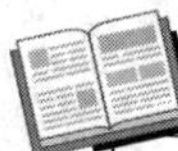

学习目标

知识要求：

1. **掌握** 香豆素类化合物的检识方法。
2. **熟悉** 异羟肟酸铁反应的操作。
3. **了解** 中药补骨脂的药材基源及药用部位。

能力要求：

学会采用异羟肟酸铁反应以及荧光检识中药中的香豆素类成分。

3.1.1 Introduction

The dried ripe fruit of *Psoralea corylifolia* L. is the source of Psoraleae Fructus (补骨脂). It is mainly used to treat impotence due to kidney deficiency, premature ejaculation, spermatorrhea, enuresis, cold pain of waist and knee, frequent micturition, and external use to treat vitiligo.

It contains coumarins and flavonoids, mainly psoralen (补骨脂素), isopsoralen, coryfolin (补骨脂甲素), corylifolinin (补骨脂乙素). Psoralen preparation has photosensitive effect. It is often combined with sunlight or ultraviolet irradiation to treat vitiligo.

psoralen　　　isopsoralen

3.1.2 Principles

According to the properties of lactones with high solubility in organic solvent and low solubility in water, furocoumarins (呋喃香豆素) are extracted from Psoraleae Fructus with 50% ethanol. The coumarins are obtained by decolorizing with activated charcoal.

3.1.3 Material and Reagents

Material: Psoraleae Fructus 50g.

Reference substance: psoralen.

Reagents: 50% ethanol, methanol, *n*-hexane, ethyl acetate, 1% NaOH solution, concentrate hydrochloric acid, ferric hydroxamate reagent, silica gel TLC plate.

3.1.4 Methods

(1) Extraction

Psoraleae Fructus 50g is smashed and added 200ml 50% ethanol to reflux twice, 1h for the first time, and 0.5h for the second time. Combine the solution, evaporate the ethanol until it is ethanol free, and stand overnight to make the residue ethanol volatilize. Discard the supernatant to collect the insoluble substance. It is the crude extract.

(2) Purification

Dissolve the crude extract in 30ml methanol and decolorized by adding activated charcoal and refluxing for 30min. Then filter in vacuum while the solution is hot. Cool the filtrate, needle-like crystal forms during cooling, which is crude psoralen.

(3) Identification

① Color Reaction

Ferric Hydroxamate Reaction: Take 1–2ml of sample solution, add 1–2 drops of methanol solution of hydroxylamine hydrochloride (solution a) and methanol solution of potassium hydroxide (solution b). Heat for 30min in the water bath, then add 1–2 drops of ferric chloride dissolved in 1% hydrochloric acid with concentration of 1% (w/v) (solution c). Record the phenomena.

Ring Open-Cycle Reaction: Take 1–2ml of sample solution, add 1–2 drops of 1% sodium hydroxide solution (solution a). Heat in the water bath, record the phenomenon. Then add 1–2 drops of 2% hydrochloric acid solution (solution b), and record the phenomena.

② TLC Identification

Adsorbent: Silica gel H-CMC plate.

Reference substance: psoralen.

Test solutions: MeOH solutions of the crude extract and crude psoralen.

Development solvent system: *n*-hexane-ethyl acetate (4 : 1).

Visualization: 365 nm UV light.

3.1.5 Procedure Scheme (Figure 4-6)

Psoraleae Fructus 50g
| Reflux with 200ml 50% EtOH twice (1h,0.5h)
Filtrate
| Concentrate the filtrate and remove ethanol completely
| Stand overnigtht
| Remove the supernatant
Crude extract
| Dissolve in 30ml MeOH
| Add small amount of activated charcoal
| Reflux for 30min
| Filtrate in vacuum while hot
| Crystallize with MeOH
Cude psoralen

Figure 4-6 Extraction and isolation of psoralen from Psoraleae Fructus

3.1.6 Precautions

During the concentration of 50% ethanol, ethanol with lower boiling point easily evaporate, while the remaining solution in the distillation flask consists of large amount of water with higher boiling point and small amount of ethanol. Constituents in Psoraleae Fructus with low polarity cannot dissolve in this solution, so after standing overnight they will completely precipitate. After the overnight, do not shake the solution in the flask, just discard the supernatant gently.

重点小结

中药补骨脂为豆科植物补骨脂的干燥成熟果实，含油脂较多。补骨脂中主要有效成分为香豆素类，其中补骨脂素是其代表性成分，为游离呋喃香豆素，既可溶于乙醇，也可溶于亲脂性有机溶剂，但在使用低极性有机溶剂提取时，易混入药材中的油脂等亲脂性杂质，故在此实验中选用 50% 乙醇作为提取溶剂，可去除油脂等杂质的干扰。

香豆素类化合物在紫外光灯 365nm 下具有天蓝色或蓝紫色荧光，这是该类化合物区分于其他类型成分的特殊物理性质。香豆素类化合物具有内酯结构，可发生异羟肟酸铁和开闭环反应。

本实验可分为三次（提取；脱色；检识）完成，所需总学时为 8 学时（4+2+2)。

目标检测

思考题

（1）除有机溶剂回流提取外，还可以采用哪些方法提取香豆素类化合物？

（2）香豆素的开闭环反应中，溶液由浑浊变澄清、复又变浑浊的原因？

4 Alkaloids (生物碱类)

Most of alkaloids are basic compounds biosynthesized from amino acids. So the extraction and isolation methods are always designed according to the basicity. Besides, different alkaloids and their salts have different solubility. It is also the principle of isolation alkaloids. In this section, Stephaniae Tetrandrae Radix (防己) and Coptidis Rhizoma (黄连) are taken as representative materials for introduction to the extraction, isolation and identification methods of alkaloids. And the properties of main alkaloids from Sophorae Flavescentis Radix (苦参) are introduced as the background of a designing experiment.

4.1 Extraction, Isolation and Identification of Alkaloids from Stephaniae Tetrandrae Radix

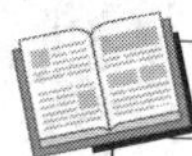

学习目标

知识要求：

1. **掌握** 生物碱的乙醇提取法、脂溶性生物碱与水溶性生物碱的分离方法。

2. **熟悉** 氧化铝柱层析分离脂溶性生物碱的方法和生物碱的检识方法；熟悉中药防己所含主要有效成分的结构特征、理化性质。

3. **了解** 防己的原植物来源及主要功效。

能力要求：

学会利用生物碱及其盐溶解度的差异设计提取分离方法；学会采用氧化铝柱层析分离脂溶性生物碱的操作方法；学会采用沉淀反应和TLC检识生物碱的方法。

4.1.1 Introduction

Stephaniae Tetrandrae Radix is the dried root of *Stephania tetrandra*. It is bitter and cold in nature. It enters the urinary bladder and lung channels. It has the effects of clearing off the wind to kill pain, resolving the water to relieve swelling. It can be used for the treatment of rheumatalgia, swelling, urinary difficulty and eczema etc. The modern pharmacological research show that the total alkaloids from Stephaniae Tetrandrae Radix have the effects of relieving pain, reducing the blood pressure, relaxing muscles and anti-inflammatory, anti-bacterial, anti-tumor activities.

Tetrandrine (粉防己碱) and fangchinoline (防己诺林碱) are the major constituents of the total alkaloids from Stephaniae Tetrandrae Radix, and the content of them should not be less than 1.6% in Stephaniae Tetrandrae Radix. Little quantity of cyclanoline (轮环藤酚碱) is also included in the total alkaloids. The main properties of these three compounds are as follows:

Tetrandrine and fangchineline are both pairs of benzyl-isoquinoline (苄基异喹啉) derivatives. Their nitrogen atoms are tertiary amine.

OMe, MeO, N, OR, H, O, O, OCH_3

tetrandrine: R = CH_3

fangchineline: R = H

Tetrandrine is colorless needle crystals. It has double melting points when it is crystallized from acetone, i.e. 126–127℃ and 217–218℃. That means it will melt at 126–127℃, then become a solid again when temperature goes up to 153℃, finally it will melt completely when the temperature goes up to 217–218℃. It is insoluble in water and petroleum ether, but it can easily dissolve in ethanol, ethyl ether, chloroform and other organic solvents and acidic aqueous solution.

Fangchineline is colorless needle-like crystals. It also has double melting points: 134–136℃ and 238–

240℃ (from acetone), 177–179℃ and 238–240℃ (from methanol). Its solubility is similar to tetrandrine, but it is more polar than tetrandrine, so the solubility in cold benzene is smaller than tetrandrine and larger in ethanol. There is a phenol hydroxyl group in frangchineline, but it is insoluble in NaOH solution.

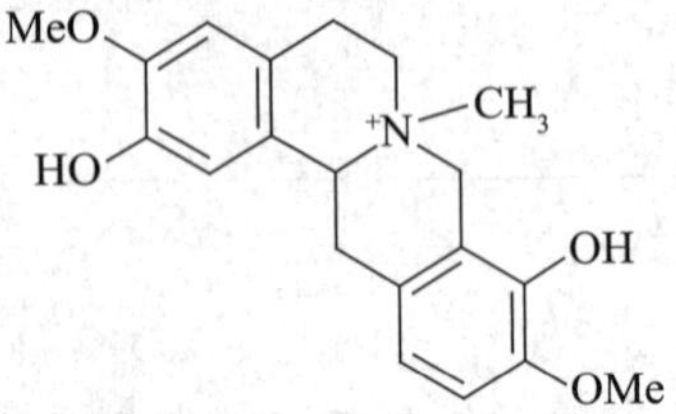

cyclanoline

Cyclanoline is water-soluble quaternary amine. It is insoluble in lipophilic organic solvents. Its chloride is colorless octahedron (八面体) -shaped crystals with melting point at 214–216℃. Its iodide is silk-like colorless crystals with melting point at 185℃. Its picrate is yellow crystals with melting point at 154–156℃.

4.1.2 Principles

Total alkaloids were extracted by reflux with ethanol, because both alkaloids and alkaloid salts are soluble in ethanol. Liposoluble and hydrosoluble alkaloids were separated by partition between lipophilic organic solvents and aqueous solution, because quaternary amines are soluble in water but insoluble in lipophilic organic solvents. Tetrandrine and fangchineline were separated by Al_2O_3 adsorption column chromatography, because fangchineline is more polar than tetrandrine. The quaternary ammonium (cyclanoline) was isolated from other water-soluble components by Reinecke salt (雷氏铵盐) precipitation.

4.1.3 Material and Reagents

Material: Powdered Stephaniae Tetrandrae Radix 100g.

Reference substances: Tetrandrine and fangchineline.

Reagents: 85%–95% EtOH, acetone, cyclohexane, ethyl acetate, hydrochloric acid, NaOH, fresh Reinecke salt, con. ammonium, 0.5% Ag_2SO_4, 10% $BaCl_2$, alkaline Al_2O_3 (100–200 mesh), pH test paper, Dragendörff reagent, Iodine-potassium iodide reagent, silicotungstic acid reagent, Wagner's reagent.

4.1.4 Methods

(1) Extraction of Total Alkaloids

Transfer 100g powder of Stephaniae Tetrandrae Radix to a 500ml round bottom flask, reflux with 85%–95% EtOH twice (300ml, 1h; 250ml, 30min), filter with cotton, combine the filtrate together and evaporate to dry, then the residue is the total extract.

(2) Separation

① Separation of Liposoluble Alkaloids and Hydrosoluble Alkaloids

Dissolve the total extract in 100ml of 1% hydrochloric acid, fully mix, filter to remove the insoluble part. Transfer the filtrate to a 500ml separatory funnel, add 70ml mixture of ethyl acetate-cyclohexane (3 : 1), drop concentrate ammonia to adjust pH to 9–10 (until no more precipitate appear in the water layer), shake to extract, release the organic layer when two layers are clear. The alkaline aqueous layer should be extracted with new mixture of ethyl acetate-cyclohexane (3 : 1) four times (50ml × 1, 40ml × 3). Combine the five times organic layers together and evaporate to dry in vacuum, the residue will be the total liposoluble alkaloids. The alkaline aqueous layer, which has been extracted by the organic mixture, should be kept for the isolation of the water-soluble alkaloid (cyclanoline).

② Separation and Purification of Hydrosoluble Alkaloid (Cyclanoline)

Filter the above alkaline aqueous layer, add 6mmol/L HCl to the filtrate to adjust the pH to 3–4, filter, add Reinecke salt saturated aqueous solution into the filtrate until the precipitate no longer generates, filter. Wash the precipitate with water, dry in the air, weigh. Dissolve the precipitate with 20times acetone, filter off the insoluble impurities, subject the acetone solution to an Al_2O_3 column (10g, dry column), elute with the mixture of acetone-water (5 : 1), collect the eluate until the color of eluate is very light. Add 0.5% Ag_2SO_4 into the eluate until no longer generating precipitate (record the volume of 0.5% Ag_2SO_4 have been used), and filter to remove the precipitate. Evaporate the filtrate to remove most of the acetone in the filtrate, cool to room temperature (filter if there is precipitate). Add 2% $BaCl_2$ solution (same moles with of Ag_2SO_4), stand a while, filter to remove the precipitate. Transfer the filtrate into an evaporating dish, concentrate to small volume (about 2–3ml) on a water bath and then transfer to a small flask, stand for crystallization. It will be cyclanoline hydrochloride. Recrystallization with H_2O if necessary (MW: 311.80 for Ag_2SO_4; 203.25 for $BaCl_2$).

③ Separation of Tetrandrine and Fangchineline

Adsorbent: Alkaline Al_2O_3 (100–200 mesh, Grade Ⅱ – Ⅲ) 20g.

Column: 2.5cm × 25cm.

Sample (dry): Weigh 200mg of the total liposoluble alkaloids and put it in a small dish, dissolve with acetone, add Al_2O_3 to adsorb all the sample solution (about 1g), stir and dry on the water bath until no acetone left in the alumina with samples.

Solvent system: Cyclohexane-acetone (3 : 1).

Packing column (wet method): Weigh 20g Al_2O_3 and transfer to a beaker, add 60ml the eluent, stir until no bubbles. Open the piston, pour the slurry into the column (with cotton on the bottom) through a funnel, the left adsorbent should use more eluent to make slurry and pour into the column again. The adsorbent will settle down in the column. Release the solvent until about 1.5cm layer is left on the top of the column bed.

Applying the sample and running the column: Pour the adsorbent with samples into the column through a funnel (the solvent layer should be enough to adsorb the adsorbent with samples), wash the samples left on the wall of the column with a little eluent. Begin to elute the column when all the samples go into the surface of the column, adjust the elute rate at 5ml/min, collect fractions in every about 30ml. Monitor the fractions with TLC and combine the same fraction with same compounds. Evaporate the solvent, and tetrandrine and fangchineline can be yielded from different fractions.

(3) Identification

① TLC identification

Adsorbent: Silica gel plate.

Reference substances: Tetrandrine and fangchineline (1mg/ml acetone solution, 1μl).

Test solutions: Fractions from column chromatography (2–4μl).

Development solvent system: $CHCl_3$-$(CH_3)_2CO$ (1 : 1), saturated for 15 minutes with ammonia before development.

Visualization: Dragendörff reagent.

② **Precipitation reactions**

Weigh the total liposoluble alkaloids about 10mg, dissolve with 5ml of 0.5% HCl, divided into 3 test tubes equally, add 1–3 drops of iodine-potassium iodide reagent, silicotungstic acid reagent and Dragendörff reagent respectively, and observe the phenomena.

4.1.5 Procedure Scheme (Figure 4-7)

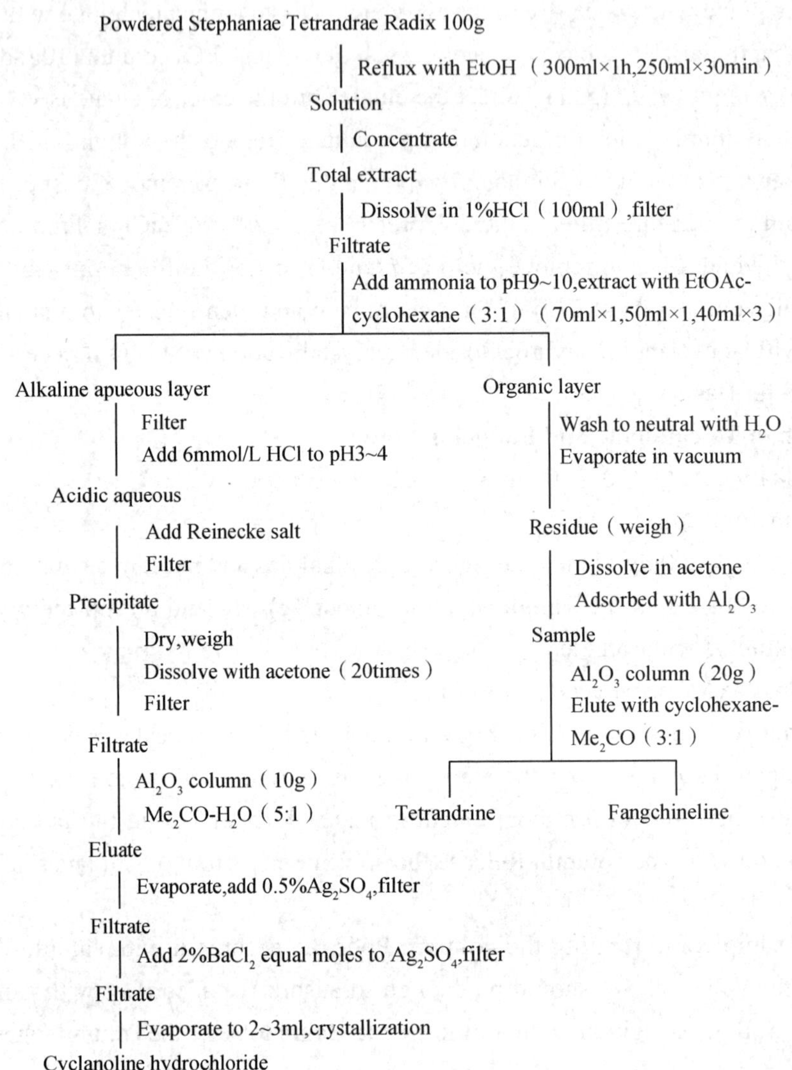

Figure 4-7 Extraction and isolation of alkaloids from Stephaniae Tetrandrae Radix

4.1.6 Precautions

(1) The organic layer for total liposoluble alkaloids should be washed to neutral by distilled water before evaporation.

(2) Enough Reinecke salt saturated aqueous solution should be added to yield complete precipitation of the water-soluble alkaloid. In the following operation, the volume of 0.5% Ag_2SO_4 solution should be recorded.

重点小结

防己为防己科植物粉防己的干燥根。防己脂溶性总生物碱中主要为粉防己碱（又称汉防己甲素）和防己诺林碱（又称汉防己乙素），均为双苄基异喹啉衍生物，氮原子呈叔胺状态。

本实验根据生物碱和生物碱盐都能溶于乙醇的通性，用乙醇回流提取法提取总碱；利用季铵型生物碱易溶于水，不溶于亲脂性有机溶剂的性质用亲脂性有机溶剂萃取法分离脂溶性生物碱和水溶性生物碱；利用粉防己碱和防己诺林碱极性的差别，用氧化铝吸附柱色谱使二者得到分离；利用季铵型生物碱与雷氏铵盐产生沉淀的性质使其与其他水溶性成分分离。

本实验可以分为三次（提取；脂溶性总生物碱和水溶性生物碱的分离以及水溶性生物碱的分离；脂溶性生物碱的分离及检识）完成。

目标检测

思考题

（1）怎样防止乳化，怎样消除乳化？

（2）一般情况下为什么有机溶剂萃取液必须洗至中性方能浓缩或放置？

（3）防己中各种生物碱的分离原理是什么？

（4）雷氏铵盐法分离纯化季铵碱有何优缺点？雷氏铵盐使用时为什么要新鲜配制？

4.2 Extraction, Isolation and Identification of Alkaloids from Coptidis Rhizoma

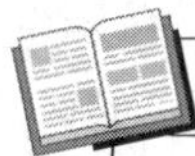

学习目标

知识要求：

1. **掌握** 水溶性生物碱的提取方法及采用制备薄层分离化合物的方法。

2. **熟悉** 生物碱的沉淀反应及小檗碱的特殊检识反应。

3. **了解** 中药黄连的药材基源及药用部位。

能力要求：

学会利用生物碱及其盐溶解度性质设计提取及分离方法；学会采用制备薄层分离化合物的方法；学会采用沉淀反应等检识生物碱的方法。

4.2.1 Introduction

The rhizomes of *Coptis chinensis* Franch. (黄连), *C. deltoidea* C. Y. Cheng et Hsiao (三角叶黄连), and *C. teeta* Wall (云连) are the sources of Coptidis Rhizoma. It has the effects of clearing away heat and dampness, eliminating fire and detoxicating. It contains alkaloids, mainly are berberine (小檗碱), palmatine (掌叶防己碱), coptisine (黄连碱). The content of berberine is the highest, up to about 10%, and it exists in Coptidis Rhizoma in the form of hydrochloride. Berberine has strong antibacterial effect, so it is widely used in clinic. Palmatine is also used as medicine, and its antibacterial effect is similar to that of berberine.

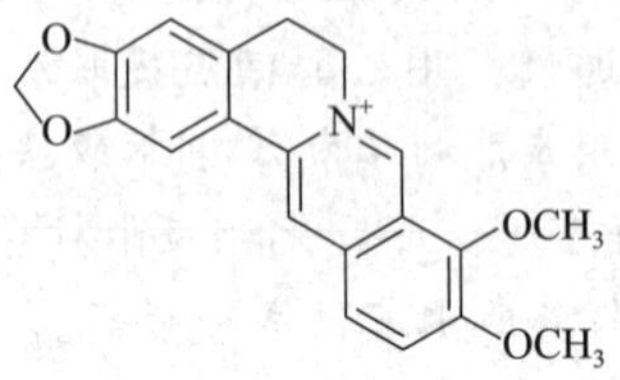

berberine 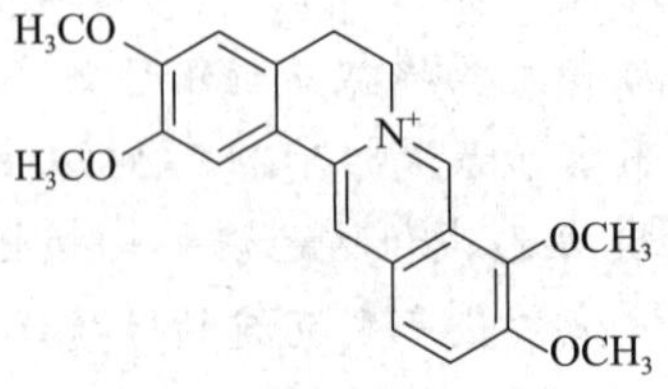　　palmatine

4.2.2 Principles

In this experiment, the total alkaloids are extracted from Coptidis Rhizoma by 0.3% sulfuric acid solution. Alkaloids with weak basicity are transferred to free form by alkalization to weak basic condition, and thus precipitate from the aqueous solution. Quaternary ammonium alkaloids such as berberine and palmatine are still soluble in the form of sulfate (1:30). Different from the sulfate of them, the hydrochlorides of berberine type alkaloids such as berberine and palmatine are hardly dissolved in water (1 : 500). By adjusting the pH value of the aqueous solution with concentrate hydrochloric acid, together with salting out with sodium chloride, berberine and palmatine precipitate in the form of hydrochlorides. Based on different polarity of berberine hydrochloride and palmatine hydrochloride, they are further separated on prepared TLC plate.

4.2.3 Material and Reagent

Material: Coptidis Rhizoma 50g.

Reference substances: berberine, palmatine.

Reagents: chloroform, methanol, glacial acetic acid, acetone, concentrated sulphuric acid, hydrochloric acid, chromotropic acid, Dragendörff reagent, silicotungstic acid reagent, calcium oxide, sodium chloride, bleaching powder, prepared and analytical silica gel TLC plate.

4.2.4 Methods

(1) Extraction of the Hydrochlorides of Berberine and Palmatine

Coptidis Rhizoma 50g is added 500ml 0.3% sulfuric acid and immersed overnight. Then the extract is collected by filter with gauze. The residue is immersed again with 300ml 0.3% sulfuric acid for 30min. Then the extract is also collected by filter with gauze. The extracts of the two immersion are combined. The pH value of the extract is adjusted with concentrate lime cream to neutral, then stand for 10min. Filter in vacuum to get the filtrate. Then the pH value of the filtrate is adjusted to 2–3 with hydrochloric acid. Sodium chloride is added according to the volume of the filtrate with the percentage 4%–5% (w/v), then stand for 10min. Filter in vacuum to get the precipitate, i.e. hydrochlorides of berberine and palmatine.

(2) Isolation of the Hydrochlorides of Berberine and Palmatine

Dissolve the precipitate in ethanol to get sample solution. Then apply the sample solution on prepared TLC plate to do isolation.

Adsorbent: prepared Silica gel H-CMC plate (20cm × 20cm).

Reference substances: berberine hydrochloride, palmatine hydrochloride.

Samples: sample solution.

Development solvent system: $CHCl_3$-MeOH-glacial acetic acid (7∶1∶2).

Visualization: 365nm UV lamp.

Collect the chromatographic bands of berberine hydrochloride and palmatine hydrochloride, respectively. Put them in conical flasks with cover, add 15ml methanol, then ultrasonic extract for 30min. Filter, concentrate the filtrate to yield berberine hydrochloride and palmatine hydrochloride, respectively.

(3) Identification

① Color Reaction

a. Acetone Addition

Dissolve the sample in hot water with the concentration of 1mg/ml. Then add 10% NaOH with the ratio of 1∶25. Heat the mixture in water bath at 50℃ after well-mixing. Then add acetone with the ratio of 1∶10. Yellow crystals indicate the existence of berberine alkaloids.

b. Ecgrine Reaction

The aqueous solution of sample is added sulfuric acid to adjust the pH to 2. Heat the mixture, then add chromotropic acid (变色酸), and keep the temperature at 70–80℃ for 20min to produce the blue purple condensation product.

This reaction can be used to differentiate berberine and palmatine. Labat reaction can also be used for the same purpose.

c. Add bleaching powder (漂白粉) or chlorine (氯气) to the aqueous solution of berberine. The solution will turn cherry red.

d. Dragendörff Reaction

The aqueous solution of sample is added 1–2 drops of hydrochloric acid, then the Dragendörff reagent. Record the phenomenon.

e. Silicotungstic Acid Reaction

The aqueous solution of sample is added 1–2 drops of hydrochloric acid, then silicotungstic acid reagent. Record the phenomenon.

② TLC Identification

Adsorbent: Silica gel H-CMC plate.

Reference substances: berberine hydrochloride, palmatine hydrochloride.

Samples: sample solution.

Development solvent system: $CHCl_3$-MeOH-Glacial acetic acid (7∶1∶2).

Visualization: 36 nm UV lamp, then spray Dragendörff reagent.

4.2.5 Procedure Scheme (Figure 4-8)

4.2.6 Precautions

(1) In the process of immersing, sulfuric acid is applied instead of hydrochloric acid for the solubility of sulfate is larger than hydrochloride for most alkaloids.

(2) The purpose of adding hydrochloric acid is to convert the sulfate of berberine and palmatine into hydrochloride, reduce their solubility in water. And the purpose of adding sodium chloride is to let the hydrochlorides precipitate completely.

(3) The desorption of samples from silica gel is achieved by ultrasonic extraction with methanol in this experiment. Successive reflux method or reflux method can also be used.

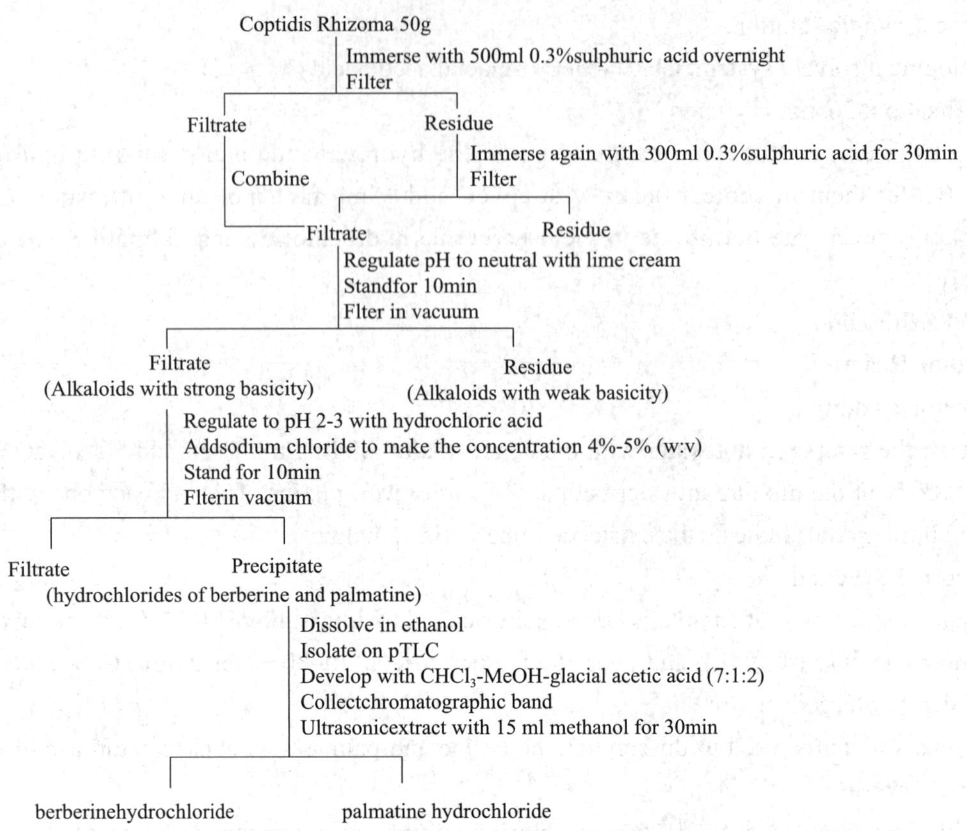

Figure 4-8 Extraction and isolation of alkaloids from Coptidis Rhizoma

重 点 小 结

中药黄连为毛茛科植物黄连、三角叶黄连和云连的干燥根茎。黄连中主要有效成分为生物碱类，小檗碱（黄连素）和掌叶防己碱是主要代表性成分。本实验首先利用生物碱的碱性差异将黄连中小檗碱和掌叶防己碱等强碱性季铵型生物碱与其他弱碱性生物碱分开，再利用小檗碱和掌叶防己碱的盐酸盐在水中溶解度低的性质将其转化为盐酸盐的形式从提取液中沉淀出来。

小檗碱和掌叶防己碱具有较长的共轭体系，在紫外灯365nm下具有黄色荧光，可用于制备薄层中色谱带的定位。小檗碱型生物碱除可发生生物碱沉淀反应外，还可以与丙酮加成产生黄色结晶、与漂白粉显色等，均可用于检识；此外，由于小檗碱结构中含有亚甲二氧基，还可以发生Ecgrine反应和Labat反应。

本实验可分为三次（提取；小檗碱和掌叶防己碱盐酸盐的分离；检识）完成。

目 标 检 测

思考题

（1）是否可用盐酸代替硫酸从黄连中提取小檗碱？

（2）实验中加入氯化钠的作用是什么？

4.3 Extraction, Isolation and Identification of Alkaloids from Sophorae Flavescentis Radix (Designing experiment)

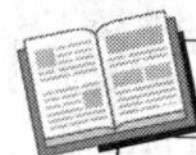

学习目标

知识要求:

1. **掌握** 生物碱的提取分离原理及常规检识方法。
2. **熟悉** 生物碱的沉淀反应。
3. **了解** 中药苦参的药材基源及药用部位。

能力要求:

学会运用中药化学成分的理化性质设计提取分离方法。

4.3.1 Introduction

The roots of *Sophora flavescens* Ait. (苦参) is the source of Sophorae Flavescentis Radix. It has the effects of clearing away heat and dampness, and is used as insecticide and diuretic. It mainly contains alkaloids and flavonoids, which are the effective constituents of it. The alkaloids in Sophorae Flavescentis Radix belong to quinolizidine (喹诺里西啶), i.e. matrine (苦参碱), oxymatrine (氧化苦参碱), etc. Matrine has the antipyretic action, analgesia, anti-convulsion and nerve stabilization effects, etc. It has obvious positive inotropic effect on cardiovascular system and can prevent and treat atherosclerosis, reduce myocardial injury, etc. It also has the functions of anti-liver injury, anti-fibrosis, increasing leukocyte, anti-tumor etc. Oxymatrine is used to treat leukopenia and chronic hepatitis, prevent liver fibrosis and cirrhosis, and has anti-arrhythmia, cardiotonic and anti-asthmatic effects.

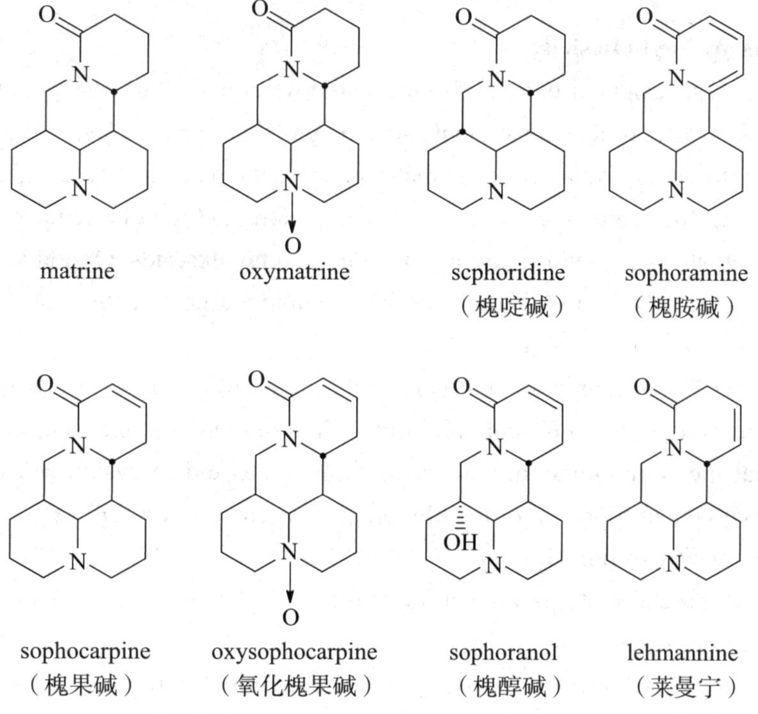

4.3.2 Physical Properties of Matrine and Oxymatrine

The physical properties of matrine and oxymatrine are listed in Table 4-2.

Table 4-2 Physical properties of matrine and oxymatrine

Compounds	Molecular formula	Melting point (°C)	Specific optical rotation	Solubility
matrine	$C_{15}H_{24}N_2O$	76	+39.11°	Soluble in methanol, ethanol, chloroform, ethyl ether Insoluble in water
oxymatrine	$C_{15}H_{24}N_2O_2$	207–208	+47.7°	Soluble in water, methanol, ethanol, chloroform Insoluble in ethyl ether

4.3.3 Requirement of Experimental Design

According to the physical properties of matrine and oxymatrine, design an experiment to extract and isolate them from Sophorae Flavescentis Radix and identify them.

4.3.4 Reference methods

(1) Extraction

① Extraction with acidic water

Dilute sulphuric acid solution can be applied to the extraction of matrine and oxymatrine. And the extraction method can be immersion, percolation, and decoction.

② Extraction with alcohol

Methanol and ethanol can be applied to the extraction of matrine and oxymatrine. And the extraction method can be immersion, percolation, refluxing, and successive refluxing. After the extraction, the solvent can be evaporated in vaccum or under atmosphere pressure.

③ Extraction with chloroform

After alkalization with ammonia, Sophorae Flavescentis Radix can be refluxed or successive refluxed with chloroform.

(2) Isolation

① Isolation according to basicity

Cation exchange resin can be used to purify the acidic water extract of Sophorae Flavescentis Radix, since there are always water soluble constituents such as proteins, saccharides, polypeptides, etc. Before subject the extract to the cation exchange resin, make sure that the resin is H-type. After the exchange, the alkali solution (such as 10% ammonia) is used for alkalization, and then organic solvents such as ethyl ether, chloroform, methanol are used for elution to yield the total alkaloids. Or add acid water or alkaline ethanol to elute the resin to obtain alkaloid salts or free alkaloids respectively.

② Isolation according to solubility

The crude extract from organic solvent can be dissolved in chloroform. Then after adding large amount of ethyl ether, due to the different solubility of matrine and oxymatrine, matrine is still in the solution, but oxymatrine is precipitated. Collect the precipitate and recrystallized with acetone to get oxymatrine. While with the evaporation of the filtrate, matrine can also crystallize.

③ Isolation according to polarity

a. Silica gel column chromatography can be applied for the isolation of matrine and oxymatrine. The solvent system can be screened by TLC.

b. Prepared silica gel TLC can also be applied for the isolation of matrine and oxymatrine.

c. Prepared HPLC with C_{18} column can be applied to isolate matrine and oxymatrine. Due to the basicity of the sample, ammonia or triethylamine is added in the mobile phase to reduce tailing. The chromophore in matrine and oxymatrine is carbonyl group, so the detection wavelength is set at 220nm.

(3) Identification

① Precipitation reactions

Use Dragendorff reagent, silicotungstic acid reagent, picric acid (苦味酸) reagent to identify them.

② TLC

Both soft plate and hard plate can be used. The adsorbent for soft plate is alumina, and that for hard plate is silica gel. Special attention should be paid when developing and visualizing the soft plate. Near horizontal development is applied. Spraying indirectly to the plate, visualizing with iodine vapor, pressing plate, or side sucking are used to visualize the soft plate.

重 点 小 结

中药苦参为豆科植物苦参的干燥根。苦参中主要有效成分为生物碱类和黄酮类，苦参碱和氧化苦参碱是主要的生物碱。实验设计中，可以利用苦参碱和氧化苦参碱的溶解度性质设计其提取方法；此外苦参碱和氧化苦参碱具有内酰胺结构，也可采用碱提 - 酸沉法。苦参碱和氧化苦参碱溶解性、碱性、极性均有差异，可利用这些差异设计分离方法。

本实验包括设计实验、准备实验材料、进行实验、结果检测等内容，所需总学时约 16 学时。

目 标 检 测

思考题

（1）选择哪种方法从苦参中提取苦参碱和氧化苦参碱？为什么？

（2）选择哪种方法分离苦参碱和氧化苦参碱？为什么？

5 Saponins (皂苷类)

Saponins are a group of glycosides. According to the sapogenin, saponins are classified into triterpenoid saponins and steroidal saponins. Saponins consist of polycyclic aglycones attached to one or more sugar side chains. Due to their structural diversities, including different types of aglycones and the numbers and types of sugar chains attached to aglycones, extraction and isolation of saponins pose a great challenge to us. Generally speaking, saponins are highly polar and water or dilute alcohol is popular to extract saponins. *n*-Butanol is generally used to extract saponins from aqueous solution. Some of triterpenoid saponins are acidic due to substituting with carboxyl group. Acidic saponins need special

strategy to do extraction and isolation. Here, Glycyrrhizae Radix et Rhizoma is selected as representative material for introduction to the extraction, isolation and identification methods of saponins.

Extraction, Isolation and Identification of Saponins from Glycyrrhizae Radix et Rhizoma

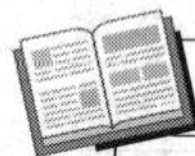

学习目标

知识要求：

1. **掌握** 皂苷类成分的理化性质和提取分离方法的原理。
2. **熟悉** 皂苷类成分的结构特点和检识方法。
3. **了解** 皂苷类成分的结构类型、分布情况和生物活性。

能力要求：

学会利用三萜皂苷的性质设计提取分离及检识方法，学会三萜皂苷常用的水解方法。

5.1.1 Introduction

Glycyrrhizae Radix et Rhizoma is the dried root and rhizome of *Glycyrrhiza uralensis* Fisch. (甘草), *G. inflate* Bat. (胀果甘草), or *G. glabra* L. (光果甘草). It is collected in spring or autumn, removed from rootlet, and dried in the air. It is used in hypofunction of the spleen and the stomach marked by lassitude and weakness; cardiac palpitation and shortness of breath; cough with much phlegm; spasmodic pain in the epigastrium, abdomen and limbs; carbuncles and sores, also used for reducing the toxic or drastic actions of other drugs. The main constituent is glycyrrhizin (甘草皂苷), which belongs to triterpenoid saponin and is composed of glycyrrhetinic acid (甘草次酸) and two glucuronic acids.

Glycyrrhizin, also named glycyrrhizic acid (甘草酸), is colorless columnar crystal, with melting point 220℃ (decomposition) and $[\alpha]_D^{27}$ +46.2°. Glycyrrhizin is a polar compound, and easily dissolve in hot dilute alcohol and dilute ammonium aqueous, not soluble in alcohol or ethyl ether. In General, glycyrrhizin is presented as potassium or calcium salt in plant. Its water solution exhibits weak foaming and hemolysis function. It has diversified activities, such as anti-virus, anti-tumor, immune modulation, detoxification, glucocorticoid action and free radical scavenging, etc.

COOH
O
glcA —O
2
glcA

glycyrrhizin

Glycyrrhetinic acid is the sapogenin of glycyrrhizic acid, after removing of two glucuronic acids (glc A) in hydrolysis. Based on the chemical structure, glycyrrhetinic acid belongs to pentacyclic triterpenes.

There are two types of glycyrrhetinic acid. One is that the configuration of D/E ring is *cis* fused (i.e., 18β-H), needle crystals, with melting point at 256℃, $[\alpha]_D^{20}$ +86°(ethanol). The other is its isomer, the D/E ring is *trans* fused, 18-α-glycyrrhetinic acid, also known as uralenic acid (乌拉尔甘草次酸), small flaky crystals, with melting point 283℃, $[\alpha]_D^{20}$ +140°(ethanol). The two crystals are both soluble in ethanol or chloroform. Glycyrrhetinic acid (18β-H) has the following activities as anti-inflammation, anti-ulcer, anti-allergy, antitussive, anti-asthmatic, expectorant, hypolipidemic, hepatic protection, and liver cancer inhibition.

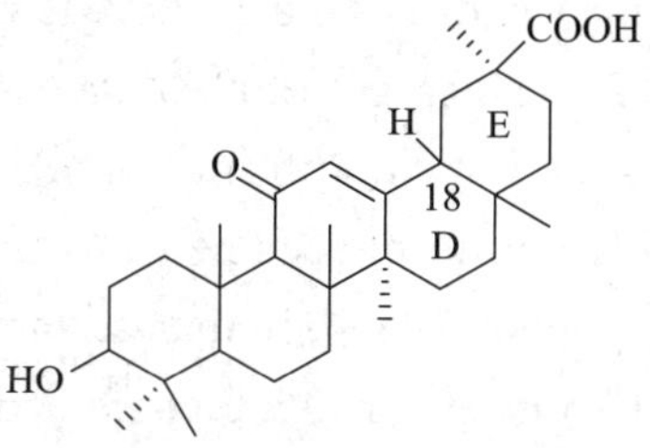

COOH
H E
O
18
D
HO

glycyrrhetinic acid

5.1.2 Principles

As mentioned in the introduction, glycyrrhizin is usually formed as salt with potassium or calcium in plant. So, glycyrrhizin can be easily precipitated by acid from the water extract solution. As it can dissolve in acetone, the crude glycyrrhizin can be firstly purified through acetone extraction. Using the acidity of glycyrrhizin, it can react with KOH to produce tripotassium glycyrrhizinate which can offer monopotassium glycyrrhizinate through purification in acetic acid. Monopotassium glycyrrhizinate can be hydrolyzed in the presence of 5% H_2SO_4 to yield glycyrrhetinic acid which can be purified through silica gel column chromatography.

5.1.3 Material and Reagents

Material: Glycyrrhizae Radix et Rhizoma extract 200g.

Reference substances: glycyrrhetinic acid.

Reagents: dilute sulfuric acid, 20% KOH/EtOH solution, acetic acid, 95% EtOH solution, silica gel (200–300 mesh), chloroform, acetone, cyclohexane, ethyl acetate, $SbCl_3/CHCl_3$ solution.

5.1.4 Methods

(1) Preparation of Crude Glycyrrhizin

Glycyrrhizae Radix et Rhizoma extract (200g) is dissolved in 4000ml distilled water, and diluted sulfuric acid is added dropwise to adjust pH 2–3 with stirring to yield a lot of brown precipitate. Through filtration, the brown precipitate (crude glycyrrhizin) is obtained. Wash to neutral with distilled water and dry.

(2) Preparation of Crude Glycyrrhetinic Acid

① Crude glycyrrhizin is grinded to powder, refluxing with acetone three times (2h, 1h, and 1h, respectively), and filter when the extract solution is still warm. The warm filtrate is cooled, and 20% KOH/EtOH solution is added to adjust pH 7–8 to produce a lot of brown-red powder precipitate. Filter to collect the precipitate, dry at room temperature, then it is crude tripotassium glycyrrhizinate.

② Crude tripotassium glycyrrhizinate is grinded, two times of quantity acetic acid are added, and the mixture is warmed till complete dissolution. The solution is stored at room temperature for 24h to recrystallize. The recrystallized solid is filtered and wash with 95% EtOH solution. Then monopotassium glycyrrhizinate is obtained.

③ Monopotassium glycyrrhizinate (3g) is moved to a 100ml round bottom flask, 5% sulfuric acid (30ml) is added, and refluxing for 1.5h to hydrolyze. The mixture is cooled to room temperature and filtered. The precipitate is washed to neutral with distilled water, and dried to yield crude glycyrrhetinic acid.

(3) Purification of Glycyrrhetinic Acid

Crude glycyrrhetinic acid (200mg) is dissolved in EtOH, mixed with silica gel, evaporated to remove the solvent, grinded, packed onto silica gel (200–300mesh) column chromatography (2.5cm × 50cm), and eluted with gradient solvents, i.e. chloroform (50ml), chloroform-acetone (10 : 1) 100ml, chloroform-acetone (8 : 1) 100ml, and chloroform-acetone (6 : 1) 100ml. Low pressure (0.3–0.5kg/cm^2) is added to accelerate the elution. The fraction is collected and examined through TLC identification. The fractions showing the same color spot with reference are combined and concentrated, and the residue is recrystallized with dilute EtOH solution to yield pure glycyrrhetinic acid.

(4) Identifications

① TLC Identification

Adsorbent: Silica gel GF_{254} plate.

Reference substances: Glycyrrhetinic acid (1mg/ml acetone solution, 2μl).

Test solutions: Fractions from silica gel column chromatography (2–4μl).

Development solvent system: cyclohexane-ethyl acetate-acetic acid (3 : 1 : 0.2).

Visualization: $SbCl_3/CHCl_3$ solution.

② Melting Point Detection

To determine the melting point, and check the literature values.

5.1.5 Procedure scheme (Figure 4-9)

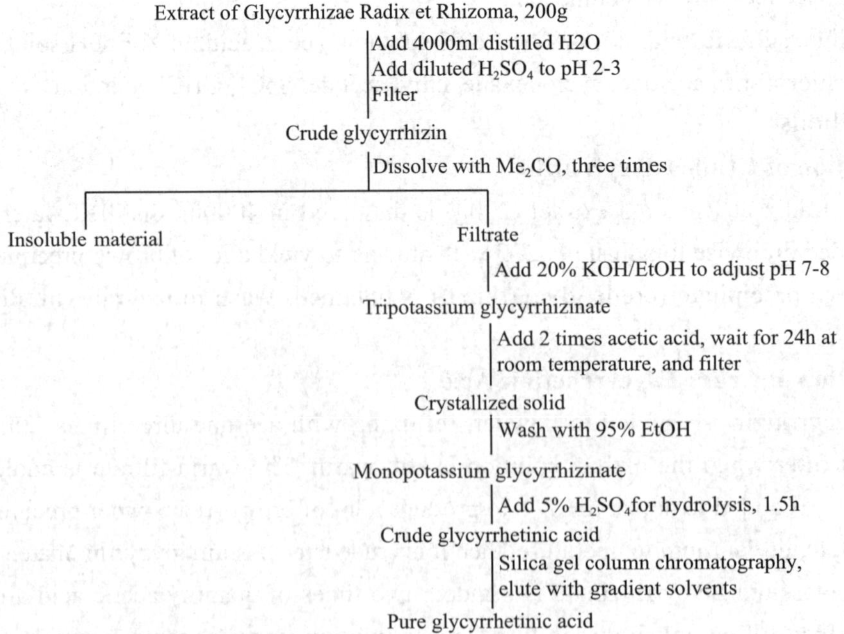

Figure 4-9 Preparation of glycyrrhetinic acid from Glycyrrhizae Radix et Rhizoma extract

5.1.6 Precautions

Please pay attention to steady and seal the column when using low-pressure column, and prevent the pressure getting too low.

重点小结

甘草为豆科植物甘草、胀果甘草或光果甘草的干燥根及根茎。甘草中的主要有效成分是甘草皂苷（又称甘草酸）和甘草次酸，还含有乌拉尔甘草皂苷A、B及多种游离的三萜类化合物和黄酮类化合物。

本实验利用甘草皂苷以钾盐或钙盐形式存在于甘草中，易溶于水，于水溶液中加酸酸化，即可析出游离的甘草皂苷（总皂苷）；利用总皂苷的极性，用丙酮溶解，除去不溶物；利用甘草酸的酸性，可与KOH生成甘草酸三钾盐，该三钾盐在乙酸纯化后得到甘草酸单钾盐；甘草酸单钾盐在5%硫酸溶液中回流水解得到甘草次酸粗品；利用甘草次酸的极性，进行硅胶柱色谱分离纯化，得到甘草次酸的纯品。

本实验可分为两次（甘草酸单钾盐的制备；甘草次酸的制备）完成。

目标检测

思考题

（1）甘草总皂苷的提取原理是什么？皂苷还有哪些提取分离方法？
（2）如何判断甘草酸单钾盐是否水解完全？为什么？

6 Volatile oils（挥发油）

Volatile oils (essential oils) are oily liquid present in plants possessing volatility, distillable with steam and water insoluble. They can evaporate when exposed to the air at room temperature. In chemistry, monoterpenoids and sesquiterpenoids are the main components of volatile oils. In this section, Menthae Haplocalycis Herba (薄荷) is taken as a representative material for introduction to the extraction and identification of volatile oils.

Extraction and Identification of Volatile Oils from Menthae Haplocalycis Herba

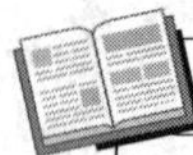

学习目标

知识要求:

1. **掌握** 挥发油的理化性质和提取方法。
2. **熟悉** 挥发油的检识和定性分析方法。
3. **了解** 薄荷挥发油的生物活性。

能力要求:

学会采用水蒸气蒸馏法从中药中提取挥发油;学会挥发油的检识和定性分析方法。

6.1.1 Introduction

Menthae Haplocalycis Herba is the dry aerial part of *Mentha haplocalyx* Briq. (薄荷). It can expel wind-heat from the head and eyes and promote eruptions. So, it can be used for the indications of headache in influenza, upper respiratory infection and other epidemic febrile diseases at the initial stage; inflammation of eyes, sore throat, ulcers in the mouth; rubella measles; discomfort and distension in the chest and hypochondriac regions. The main constituents in volatile oils (contents > 0.8%) from Menthae Haplocalycis Herba include menthol, menthone and menthyl acetate. Meanwhile, Menthae Haplocalycis Herba also contains flavonoids such as menthosides, isoraifolin, etc.

6.1.2 Principles

Volatile oils are immiscible with water. When the total pressure of volatile oils and water steam equals with atmospheric pressure under heating, the solution starts to boil and distills if heated continually. So, the volatile oils can be extracted with steam distillation method and the content of volatile oil can be determined by this method.

6.1.3 Material and Reagents

Material: Menthae Haplocalycis Herba 200g.

Reagents: sodium chloride, vanillin-H_2SO_4 solution.

6.1.4 Methods

(1) Extraction of Spearmint Oil (薄荷油)

Menthae Haplocalycis Herba (200g) is moved to a 1000ml round bottom flask, 500ml distilled water is added, and mixed completely. The flask is then connected with volatile oil extractor (挥发油提取器, the type of that oil is lighter than water), and distilled water is added to scale division of the determinant until water overflow back to the flask. The mixture is heated slightly by an electric jacket to boil for about 5h until the quantity of the oil does not increase. After that, the piston at the bottom of the extractor is opened so that water can flow out until upper surface of oil layer reach to 5mm above the zero-degree line. One hour later, the piston is opened again so that the top of oil layer reach zero-degree line. The quantity of oil is read through the scale, and the content percentage of oil in raw material is calculated herein.

(2) Identification of Spearmint Oil

① Physical Constants Determination

a. Relative density

$$d_{t_1}^{t_2} = \frac{w_2}{w_1}$$

t_1: temperature of water; t_2: temperature of spearmint oil; w_1: weight of water; w_2: weight of Spearmint oil; d: relative density of Spearmint oil.

b. Refractive index

Use a refractometer read the refractive index (n_D^t).

n: refractive index; D: sodium light; t: temperature of determining

c. Optical rotation

Use a polarimeter to detect the optical rotation and calculate by following equation:

$$[a]_D^t = \frac{100a}{L \times C}$$

$[\alpha]$: optical rotation; D: sodium light; t: temperature of determining; α: count of the polarimeter; L: length of sample tube (unit as decimeter); C: gram of sample in 100ml.

② TLC Identification

Adsorbent: silica gel plate.

Sample: spearmint oil.

Development solvent system: petroleum ether-ethyl acetate (85 : 15).

Visualization: vanillin-H_2SO_4 solution.

6.1.5 Precautions

(1) Adding sodium chloride can improve speed of distilling and shorten time of distilling.

(2) According to the relative density, choose the correct quantitative test method and Extractor.

重点小结

薄荷为唇形科植物薄荷的干燥地上部分，含有较多的挥发油，挥发油里的主要成分包括薄荷醇、薄荷酮、醋酸薄荷酮等；薄荷除了挥发油还含有黄酮类等成分。本实验利用薄荷油与水不互溶，在水中受热后，二者蒸气压的总和与大气压相等时，溶液即开始沸腾，继续加热则薄荷油可随水蒸气蒸馏出来。因此，薄荷中的挥发油可采取水蒸气蒸馏法来提取，并进行物理常数的测定（包括密度、折光率和比旋光度）和薄层检识等定性分析。

本实验可分为两次（提取；检识）完成，所需总学时为 10 学时（6+4)。

目标检测

思考题

（1）挥发油的通性有哪些？应如何保存？
（2）简述挥发油的化学组成及主要功能基团。
（3）挥发油类成分常用的定性方法有哪些？

题库

Reference Answers to Object Detections
目标检测参考答案

第二章

（1）中药化学成分主要通过溶剂法进行提取，该方法中包括两部分：一是根据中药化学成分的溶解性和酸碱性选择适宜的提取溶剂；二是根据中药材的性质、中药化学成分的稳定性等选择适宜的提取方式。提取溶剂的选择主要依据“相似相溶”的原理。提取方式则分为浸渍、渗漉、煎煮、回流和连续回流提取法，对于热不稳定的化学成分多采用浸渍和渗漉等冷提取方式，溶剂常选用极性较大、渗透力强的溶剂；对于热稳定的化学成分，为提高提取效率则常采用煎煮、回流和连续回流等热提取方式。此外，中药中的挥发性成分常采用水蒸气蒸馏法进行提取。

（2）用石油醚萃取可获得油脂、蜡、叶绿素、挥发油、游离甾体及三萜类化合物，用三氯甲烷或乙酸乙酯可获得游离生物碱、有机酸及黄酮、香豆素的苷元等中等极性化合物，用正丁醇萃取可获得苷类、生物碱盐以及鞣质等极性化合物，剩余的水层中可能含有氨基酸、糖类、无机盐等水溶性成分。

（3）选择适宜的溶剂对于结晶法是否成功至关重要。首先，所选溶剂不得与待纯化成分起化学反应，通常在高温度时对待纯化成分溶解度大、温度降低时溶解度降低。其次，所选溶剂对杂质的溶解度非常大或非常小，前一种情况有利于杂质留存在母液中，后一种情况有利于通过趁热抽滤的操作除去杂质。最后，溶剂的沸点不宜过高、也不宜过低，高沸点溶剂易附着于结晶表面，低沸点溶剂制成溶液和冷却析晶的温差小、操作不便。

（4）柱色谱法根据其分离原理可分为吸附柱色谱、分配柱色谱、离子交换色谱和排阻色谱。

第三章

（1）该药材的石油醚提取物 Liebermann–Burchard 反应阳性提示其可能含有三萜或甾体苷元，与溴麝香草酚蓝、三氯化铁试剂显色提示其可能含有羧酸、酚类。乙醇提取物可发生 Molish 反应提示其含有糖或苷类，可发生 HCl–Mg 反应提示其含有黄酮类化合物。与碘化铋钾、硅钨酸和苦味酸等生物碱沉淀试剂生成沉淀说明可能存在生物碱。水提取物可发生 Molish 反应提示其含有糖类，与雷氏铵盐生成沉淀提示可能含有季铵型生物碱。

（2）分别以石油醚、乙醇和水提取山楂药材。分别测试其是否可与 Liebermann–Burchard、Molish、HCl–Mg 等发生阳性反应，以及是否与溴麝香草酚蓝、三氯化铁、明胶等试剂发生阳性反应，从而推断出其含有的化合物结构类型。山楂中含有黄酮（苷）、有机酸、鞣质、三萜等类型化合物，以上反应均为阳性。

第四章

1.1 参考答案

（1）根据虎杖中游离蒽醌结构中酚羟基数目和位置（α- 酚羟基由于可与相邻的羰基形成分子内氢键，其酸性弱于 β- 酚羟基）有不同强度的酸性，用碱性强度递增的水溶液（5% $NaHCO_3$，5% Na_2CO_3，2% NaOH）自有机溶剂中分别萃取出不同酸性强弱的游离蒽醌类成分，分离后再分别酸化，得到游离蒽醌。

（2）大黄酚结构中仅含有两个 α- 酚羟基，酸性较弱，大黄素结构中除了两个 α- 酚羟基，还含有一个 β- 酚羟基，酸性较强；因此大黄素的极性要比大黄酚的极性大，在 TLC 展开时，大黄酚的 R_f 值要比大黄素的 R_f 值大。

（3）乙醇是两亲性溶剂，既可以与水互溶又可以与其他亲脂性有机溶剂互溶，因此在水与亲脂性有机溶剂萃取时，残存的乙醇将起到乳化剂的作用，不利于萃取分离。

（4）萃取的操作程序：①准备，选择萃取剂和被萃取溶液总体积大一倍以上的分液漏斗，并检查分液漏斗的盖子和旋塞是否紧密（检漏）；检查的方法一般是加入一定量的水，振摇，看是否有泄露。②加料，将被萃取溶液和萃取剂分别从分液漏斗的上口倒入，并盖好盖子；必要时可使用玻璃漏斗辅助加料。萃取剂的选择要根据被萃取物质在此溶剂的溶解度而定，同时要易于和溶质分离开，最好选用低沸点溶剂；一般水溶性较小的物质可用石油醚萃取，水溶性较大的可用苯或乙醚萃取，水溶性极大的可用乙酸乙酯萃取。③振荡，分液漏斗倾斜使上口略微朝下，振摇分液漏斗使两相溶液充分接触，振摇过程中要防止漏液。④放气，振荡后让分液漏斗保持倾斜状态，打开旋塞，放出蒸气或产生的气体，使内外压力平衡；注意放气时分液漏斗的上口要倾斜朝下，而下口不要有液体。⑤重复振荡和放气。⑥将分液漏斗放在合适的铁圈上静置等待分层。若有乳化现象，可采取破乳操作。⑦分液，打开旋塞将下层液体放出，上层液体从上口倒出；如果上层液体也从旋塞放出，则漏斗旋塞下面附着的残液将污染上层液体。⑧重复萃取操作两到三次，并合并萃取液。

1.2 参考答案

（1）大黄中的化学成分多为羟基蒽醌，具有酸性，可采用碱提酸沉法进行提取。

（2）含有多个斑点的样品为混合物，可选用柱色谱分离的方法对其进行分离纯化。如本实验既采用硅胶柱色谱法，还可采用聚酰胺作为吸附剂对羟基蒽醌类化合物进行分离。

（3）蒽醌类化合物除可以发生 Bornträger 反应、金属离子络合反应、强酸显色以外，还可以发生 Feigl 反应。此外，其结构中的酚羟基也可与三氯化铁 – 铁氰化钾显色。

2 参考答案

（1）除利用黄酮类化合物的酸性采用碱提酸沉法提取黄酮类化合物外，还可以利用相似相溶法，以水或乙醇等作为提取溶剂，采用煎煮法或回流法提取黄酮类化合物。

（2）除结晶法外，还有水提醇沉法、醇提水沉法、醇 – 醚法、醇 – 丙酮法、碱 – 酸法、酸 – 碱法等利用物质的溶解度差异进行分离的操作，其中前四种是通过改变溶剂的极性从而改变物质的溶解度，后两种是通过改变物质的存在状态（离解 – 游离）从而改变物质的溶解度。

（3）芦丁酸水解过程中水解液由浑浊变澄清、复又浑浊的原因：加入酸水时，芦丁因在室温下在水中溶解度低，故而浑浊；加热回流进行后，溶液温度升高，芦丁溶解度升高，因而澄清；水解反应开始后，芦丁被酸水解生成槲皮素，槲皮素在水中溶解度低，因此溶液最终又变浑浊。

3 参考答案

（1）除利用相似相溶法，以乙醇等作为提取溶剂，采用回流法提取香豆素类化合物外，还可利用香豆素化合物的内酯采用碱溶酸沉法提取香豆素类化合物。

（2）开闭环反应中，在样品的甲醇溶液中加入氢氧化钠溶液后，由于溶剂极性增大，补骨脂素等香豆素类成分溶解度减小，因而溶液浑浊；置于水浴加热后，香豆素的内酯环开环生成顺式邻羟基桂皮酸盐的结构，溶于水，故溶液变澄清；加入盐酸后，香豆素又重新环合为内酯结构，溶解度降低，所以溶液复又浑浊。

4.1 参考答案

（1）预防乳化：可以将提取液慢慢地加入被提取液中，或只是轻轻地旋荡，乳化的倾向是能被抑制的；当发现被提溶液中存在悬浮固体时，最好在提取之前就加以过滤。

消除乳化有以下几种方法：① 长时间静置。② 水平旋转摇动分液漏斗；当两液层由于乳化而形成界面不清时，可将分液漏斗在水平方向上缓慢地旋转摇动，这样可以消除界面处的“泡沫”，促进分层。③ 用滤纸过滤；对于由于有树脂状、黏液状悬浮物存在而引起的乳化现象，可将分液漏斗中的物料，用质地密致的滤纸，进行减压过滤，过滤后物料则容易分层和分离。④ 离心分离；将乳化混合物移入离心分离机中，进行高速离心分离。⑤ 用电吹风加热乳化层。⑥ 加饱和食盐水。

（2）若为酸性有机溶剂，可中和生物碱，提取产率下降；若为碱性有机溶剂，可能发生强碱置换弱碱的反应，消耗生物碱或产生其他碱，不利于提取实验。所以要求有机溶剂必须洗至中性。

（3）根据大多数生物碱或生物碱盐都能溶于乙醇的通性，用乙醇回流提取法提取总碱；利用季铵型生物碱易溶于水，不溶于亲脂性有机溶剂的性质用溶剂萃取法分离脂溶性生物碱和水溶性生物碱；利用粉防己碱和防己诺林碱极性的差别，用氧化铝吸附柱色谱法使二者得到分离；利用季铵型生物碱与雷氏铵盐产生沉淀的性质使其与其他水溶性成分分离。

（4）雷氏铵盐法优点为选择性沉淀分离季铵生物碱，专属性强，分离效率高，缺点为价格昂贵，不宜工业化生产。雷氏铵盐为 Cr 与氨分子及 SCN^- 的络合物，久置易分解，故应现用现制。

4.2 参考答案

（1）生物碱含氧酸盐的溶解度大于卤代酸盐，因此在以酸水作为提取溶剂提取生物碱时多采用硫酸。而小檗碱型生物碱的盐酸盐水溶性差，不利于其从药材中渗出，故本实验采用的是硫酸。

（2）实验过程中加盐酸调至 pH 2–3，该操作的目的是先将小檗碱的硫酸盐转化成盐酸盐；加滤液体积 4%–5% 的 NaCl，一方面是利用 Cl^- 的同离子效应，增加小檗碱盐酸盐的生成，另一方面是利用盐析效应，进一步降低小檗碱盐酸在水中的溶解度，从而析出沉淀。

4.3 参考答案

（1）可以根据苦参碱和氧化苦参碱具有碱性，选择酸水作为提取溶剂，采用浸渍、渗漉或者煎煮法进行提取。也可根据苦参碱和氧化苦参碱可溶于乙醇，用乙醇浸渍、渗漉、回流或连续回流提取。

（2）苦参碱和氧化苦参碱在乙醚中溶解度差异较大，其中氧化苦参碱因具有半极性的配位键，难溶于乙醚，故可以先将二者溶于三氯甲烷中，再加数倍量乙醚，氧化苦参碱即沉淀析出。此外也可采用硅胶、氧化铝柱色谱或制备液相色谱对二者进行分离。

5 参考答案

（1）甘草皂苷可以钾盐或钙盐形式存在于甘草中，易溶于水，于水溶液中加稀酸即可析出游离的甘草皂苷，经过过滤即可得总皂苷。

皂苷的提取方法有：①甲醇或乙醇提取；②酸水回流并用有机溶剂提取；③碱水提取法。

皂苷的分离方法有：①沉淀法，梯度沉淀，在醇溶液中加入丙酮或乙醚；胆固醇沉淀。②色谱分离方法，吸附色谱法，分配色谱法，HPLC 法，大孔树脂色谱法，凝胶色谱法。

（2）薄层色谱法是监测反应过程的常用方法。在本实验中可用薄层色谱检识甘草酸单钾盐是否水解完全。即取反应前的溶液及水解液点于硅胶 GF_{254} 薄层板上，以正丁醇－浓氨水－水－95% 乙醇（50∶4∶10∶10）为展开剂进行展开，展开后观察甘草酸单钾盐的斑点是否消失。如果斑点消失，证明甘草酸单钾盐被完全水解。

6 参考答案

（1）挥发油的通性有：①无色或淡黄色油状液体；②挥发性、与水不互溶、可随水蒸气蒸馏；③大多具有芳香嗅味；④大多具有光学活性；⑤可溶于醚、醇等有机溶剂；⑥不稳定，易氧化和酯化。挥发油应于棕色瓶内密闭并阴凉处保存，因为挥发油对光线、空气及温度均敏感。

（2）挥发油的主要化学成分：①萜类化合物；②芳香族小分子化合物；③脂肪族小分子化合物；④其他挥发性物质。主要功能基团有：双键、内酯环、酚羟基、醛基或酮基。

（3）挥发油类成分常用的定性方法有：①物理常数，如相对密度、折光率、比旋光度；②化学常数，如酸值、酯值、皂化值。

Appendices

附　　录

Ⅰ Frequently Used Solvents（常用溶剂）

NO.	Solvent	Polarity Index	Dielectric constants	Viscosity (20°C)	Boiling point (°C)	Solubility in water (% W/W)
1	Petroleum ether（石油醚）	0.6	1.8	0.3	30–60	0
2	Cyclohexane（环己烷）	0.6	2	1	81	0.01
3	*n*-Hexane（正己烷）	0.9	1.9	0.33	69	0.01
4	Diethyl ether（乙醚）	11.7	4.3	0.23	35	6.9
5	Ethyl acetate（乙酸乙酯）	23	6	0.45	77	8.7
6	Chloroform（三氯甲烷）	25.9	4.8	0.57	61	0.81
7	Methylene chloride（二氯甲烷）	30.9	9.1	0.44	40	1.6
8	Acetone（丙酮）	35.5	20.6	0.32	56	100
9	Acetonitrile（乙腈）	46	37.5	0.37	82	100
10	*i*-Propanol（异丙醇）	54.6	18.3	2.37	82	100
11	*n*-Butanol（正丁醇）	60.2	18.2	2.95	118	7.81
12	Acetic acid（乙酸）	64.8	6.2	1.28	118	100
13	Ethanol（乙醇）	65.4	22.4	1.2	78	100
14	Methanol（甲醇）	76.2	32.6	0.6	65	100
15	Water（水）	100	79.7	1	100	100

Ⅱ Glossary（词汇表）

A		
abscissa	[æb'sisə]	n. 横坐标
adhesive	[əd'hi:siv]	n. 黏合剂
adjuvant	['ædʒuvənt]	n. 辅助药
adsorbent	[æd'sɔ:bənt]	n. 吸附剂
alkaloid	['ælkəlɔid]	n. 生物碱
aloe-emodin	['æləu]['emədin]	芦荟大黄素
4-aminoantipyrine	[ˌæmiˌnəu][ˌænti'paiərin]	4- 氨基安替比林
ammonia	[ə'məunjə]	n. 氨水
aniline	['ænili:n]	n.（adj.）苯胺（的）
anion	['ænaiən]	n. 阴离子
anthracene	['ænθrəsi:n]	n. 蒽
anthraquinone	[ˌænθrə'kwinəun]	n. 蒽醌
antimony pentachloride	['æntiməni][pentə'klɔ:raid]	五氯化锑
applicator	['æplikeitə]	n. 涂敷器
ascending development	[ə'sendiŋ][di'veləpment]	上行展开
aurone	[au'rəunz]	n. 橙酮
azide	['æzaid]	n. 叠氮
B		
barium carbonate	['bεəriəm]['ka:bəneit]	n. 碳酸钡
benzyl isoquinoline	['benzil][ˌaisəkwai'nəli:n]	n. 苄基异喹啉
berberine	['bə:bəri:n]	n. 小檗碱
betulin	['betjulin]	n. 白桦脂醇
bismuth potassium iodide	['bizməθ][pə'tæsiəm]['aiədaid]	碘化铋钾
biuret	[bjə'ret]	n. 双缩脲
bleaching powder	['bli:tʃiŋ]['paudə]	漂白粉
boric acid	['bɔ:rik]['æsid]	硼酸
bromothymol blue	[b'rəuməθiməl]	溴麝香草酚蓝
buchner funnel	['fʌnl]	布氏漏斗

C		
caffeine	[ke'fi:n]	n. 咖啡因
casserole	['kæsərəul]	n. 砂锅
catechin	['kætitʃin]	n. 儿茶素
cation	['kætaiən]	n. 阳离子
chalcone	['kælˌkəun]	n. 查耳酮
cerium sulfate	['siəriəm]['sʌlˌfeɪt]	硫酸铈
chlorine	['klɔ:ri:n]	n. 氯气
chromotropic acid	[krəuməut'rəpik]	变色酸
chrysophanol	['krisəfənəl]	n. 大黄酚
column chromatography	['kɔləm][ˌkrəumə'tɔgrəfi]	柱色谱
condensation	[ˌkɔnden'seɪʃən]	n. 冷凝
Coptidis rhizoma	[rai'zəumə]	黄连
Coptis chinensis Franch..		黄连
Coptis deltoidea C.Y.Cheng et Hsiao		三角叶黄连
Coptis teeta Wall.		云连
coptisine	['kɔptisin]	n. 黄连碱
coryfolin	[kɔ:ri:'fəulin]	n. 补骨脂甲素
corylifolinin	[kɔ:rili'fəulinin]	n. 补骨脂乙素
coumarin	['ku:mərin]	n. 香豆素
crystallization	[kristəli'zeiʃən]	n. 结晶
cyclanoline	[sik'lænəli:n]	n. 轮环藤酚碱
D		
decoction	[di'kɔkʃən]	n. 煎煮
decolorization	[di:kʌlərai'zeiʃən]	n. 脱色
descending development	[di'sendiŋ][di'veləpm(e)nt]	下行展开
diatomite	[dai'ætəmait]	n. 硅藻土
diazotization	[daiˌæzəti'zeiʃən]	n. 重氮化
2,6-dichloroquinone-4-chloroimide	[daiklɔrəu'kwinəun klɔrəu'imaid]	2,6– 二氯苯醌氯亚胺
dihydroflavone	[daiˌhaidrə'flævənɔl]	n. 二氢黄酮
dihydroflavonol	[daiˌhaidrə'flævənɔl]	n. 二氢黄酮醇

E		
electrolyte	[iˈlektrəlait]	n. 电解质
eluate	[ˈeljuit]	n. 洗出液
eluent	[ˈeljuənt]	n. 洗脱液
emodin	[ˈemədin]	n. 大黄素
emulsification	[iˈmʌlsifikeiʃən]	n. 乳化
enamel	[iˈnæml]	n. 搪瓷
ephedrine	[eˈfedrin]	n. 麻黄碱
essential oil	[iˈsenʃl]	n. 精油
evaporating dish	[iˈvæpəreitiŋ][diʃ]	n. 蒸发皿
F		
fangchinoline	[ˈfæŋˈtʃnəlin]	n. 汉防己乙素，防己诺林碱
faucet	[ˈfɔ:sit]	n. 旋塞
ferric hydroxamate	[ˈferik][haiˈdrɔksæmət]	异羟肟酸铁
ferric trichloride	[ˈferik][traiˈklɔ:raid]	三氯化铁
filtrate	[ˈfiltreit]	n. 滤液
flavones	[ˈfleivəunz]	n. 黄酮
flavonoids	[ˈfleivənəuidz]	n. 黄酮类
flavonol	[fleivəˈnɔl]	n. 黄酮醇
freeze-dried	[fri:z][draid]	冷冻干燥
furocoumarin	[fuərəuˈkəmərin]	n. 呋喃香豆素
G		
gelatin	[ˈdʒelətin]	n. 明胶
glycyrrhetinic acid	[ˌglaisiriˈtinik][ˈæsid]	甘草次酸
Glycyrrhiza glabra L.		光果甘草
Glycyrrhiza inflata Bat		胀果甘草
Glycyrrhiza uralensis Fisch		甘草
Glycyrrhizae radix et rhizoma		甘草
glycyrrhizic acid	[ˌglisiˈraizik][ˈæsid]	甘草酸
glycyrrhizin	[gliˈkə:raizin]	n. 甘草皂苷
gypsum	[ˈdʒipsəm]	n. 石膏

H		
hydroxylamine hydrochloride	[haiˌdrɔksiləˈmi:n][ˌhaidəuˈklɔ:raid]	盐酸羟胺
I		
incremental multiple development	[iŋkrəˈmentl][ˈmʌltipl][diˈveləpment]	增量多次展开
L		
lehmannine	[lehˈmænin]	n. 莱曼宁
M		
maceration	[ˌmæsəˈreiʃən]	n. 浸渍
matrine	[meitˈri:n]	n. 苦参碱
Mentha haplocalyx Briq.		薄荷
Menthae haplocalycis herba		薄荷
menthol	[ˈmenˌθɔ:l]	n. 薄荷醇
menthone	[mentˈhəuni:]	n. 薄荷酮
multiple development	[ˈmʌltipl][diˈveləpment]	多次展开
N		
near horizontal development	[niə][hɔriˈzɔntl] [diˈveləpment]	近水平展开
ninhydrin	[ninˈhaidrin]	n.（水合）茚三酮
O		
octahedron	[ɔktəˈhi:drən]	n. 八面体
one-dimensional development	[wʌn][diˈmenʃənəl][diˈveləpment]	单向展开
optical rotation	[ˈɔptikl][rəuˈteɪʃən]	旋光度
ordinate	[ˈɔ:dinət]	n. 纵坐标
oxymatrine	[ɔkˈsimətrin]	n. 氧化苦参碱
oxysophocarpine	[ɔksaisəfəuˈkɑ:pin]	n. 氧化槐果碱
P		
palmatine	[ˈpælməti:n]	n. 掌叶防己碱
partition coefficient	[pɑ:ˈtiʃən][ˈkəuiˈfiʃnt]	分配系数
pedicel	[ˈpedisəl]	n. 花梗
percolation	[ˌpə:kəleiʃn]	n. 渗漉
pH gradient partition	[ˈgreidiənt][pɑ:ˈtiʃən]	pH 梯度萃取
phthalic acid	[ˈθælik][ˈæsid]	邻苯二甲酸

P		
physion	[ˈfiʃn]	n. 大黄素甲醚
picric acid	[ˈpikrik][ˈæsid]	苦味酸
piston	[ˈpistən]	n. 活塞
polydatin	[pəuˈlideitin]	n. 虎杖苷
Polygoni Cuspidati Rhizoma et Radix		虎杖
Polygonum cuspidatum Sieb. et Zucc		虎杖
porcelain	[ˈpɔ:səlin]	n. 瓷
pot	[pɔt]	n. 陶盆
potassium iodide	[pəˈtæsiəm][ˈaiədaid]	碘化钾
potassium sodium tartrate	[pəˈtæsiəm][ˈsəudiəm][ˈtɑ:treit]	酒石酸钾钠
pretreatment	[ˈpri:ˌtri:tmənt]	n. 前处理，预处理
Psoralea corylifolia		补骨脂
Psoraleae Fructus		补骨脂
psoralen	[ˈsɔ:rələn]	n. 补骨脂素，补骨脂内酯
Q		
quercetin	[ˈkwə:sitin]	n. 槲皮素
quinolizidine	[kwinəliˈzaidin]	n. 喹诺里西啶
R		
radius	[ˈreidiəs]	n. 半径
recrystallization	[ri:kristəliˈzeiʃən]	n. 重结晶
refluxing	[ˈri:flʌksiŋ]	n. 回流
Reinecke salt	[sɔ:lt]	雷氏铵盐
resorcinol	[riˈzɔ:sinəl]	n. 间苯二酚
resveratrol	[rezˈviəritrɔ:l]	n. 白藜芦醇
Rhei Radix et Rhizoma		大黄
rhein	[rain]	n. 大黄酸
Rheum officinale Baill.		药用大黄
Rheum palmatum L.		掌叶大黄
Rheum tanguticum Maxim. ex Balf.		唐古特大黄
rutin	[ˈru:tin]	n. 芦丁

S		
saponin	[ˈsæpənin]	n. 皂苷
sennoside	[seˈnəusaid]	n. 番泻苷
separation factor	[ˌsepəˈreiʃən]	n. 分离因子
separatory funnel	[ˈsepərətəri][ˈfʌnl]	分液漏斗
silicotungstic acid	[ˌsilikəuˈtuŋstik][ˈæsid]	硅钨酸
single test	[ˈsiŋgl][test]	单项实验法
siphone	[ˈsaifəun]	n. 虹吸
solvent precipitation	[ˈsɔlvənt][prisipiˈteiʃən]	溶剂沉淀
sophocarpine	[səufəˈkɑ:pi:n]	n. 槐果碱
Sophora japonica L.		槐
Sophora flavescens Ait.		苦参
Sophorae Flavescentis Radix		苦参
sophoradiol	[səufəreiˈdiəul]	n. 槐花二醇
Sophorae flos		槐花
Sophorae fructus	[fˈrʌktəs]	槐角
sophoramine	[ˌsɔfəˈræmi:n]	n. 槐胺碱
sophoranol	[ˌsɔfəˈrænɔl]	n. 槐醇
sophoridine	[səuˈfɔ:raidin]	n. 槐定碱
sophorin A	[səuˈfɔ:rin]	槐花米甲素
Soxhlet apparatus	[æpəˈreitəs]	索氏提取器
spacer sleeve	[ˈspeisə][sli:v]	隔套
spearmint oil	[ˈspiəmint][ɔil]	薄荷油
steam distillation	[sti:m][ˌdistəˈleiʃən]	水蒸气蒸馏
Stephania tetrandra S. Moore		粉防己
Stephaniae Tetrandrae Radix		防己
stilbenes	[sˈtilbəni:z]	n. 二苯乙烯类
successive reflux	[səkˈsesiv][ˈri:flʌks]	连续回流
supernatant	[sju:pəˈneitənt]	n. 上清液
systemic test	[siˈstemik][test]	系统实验法

T		
tannic acid	[ˈtænik][ˈæsid]	鞣酸
tetrandrine	[ˈtetrændrain]	n. 汉防己甲素，汉防己碱
thin layer chromatography	[θin][ˈleiə][ˌkrəumə'tɔgrəfi]	薄层色谱
thiocyanate	[θaiəu'saiəneit]	n. 硫氰酸盐
troxerutin	[trɔksə'ru:tin]	三羟乙基芦丁，曲克芦丁
two-dimensional development	[tu:][diˈmenʃənəl][diˈveləpment]	双向展开
U		
uralenic acid	[ˈæsid]	乌拉尔甘草次酸
urea	[juˈri:ə]	n. 尿素
V		
valence	[ˈveiləns]	n. 化合价
volatile oil	[ˈvɔlətail][ɔil]	挥发油
volatile oil extractor	[ˈvɔlətail][ɔil][iksˈtræktə]	挥发油提取器
X		
xanthydrol	[ˈzænθidrəl]	n. 呫吨氢醇
xylene	[ˈzaili:n]	n. 二甲苯
Z		
zeolite	[ˈzi:əlait]	n. 沸石
zirconium oxychloride	[zə:ˈkəuniəm]	n. 氯化氧锆

Main References
主要参考文献

1. 李永吉，彭代银．高等学校中药学类实验操作指南（中药学、药学及相关专业）[M]．北京：中国中医药出版社，2017.

2. 李医明．中药化学实验（双语版）[M]．北京：科学出版社，2009.

3. 梁敬钰．天然药物化学实验与指导[M]．北京：中国医药科技出版社，2010.